What Others Are Saying About

THE NIGHTINGALE CONSPIRACY . . .

"This book could make a great gift for any nurse - or for any nurse to give herself! Changes will soon come fast and furious in health care reform. If nursing wants to have a say (which we must) *THE NIGHTINGALE CONSPIRACY* is one major way to prepare for the paradigm shift. Finally, our big opportunity to be a powerful force in the upcoming changes, and to claim our voice at last! This book is rich with food for thought, helping each nurse to get back in touch with her own voice, her own nurse-healer, her own role as a leader in the health care revolution."
Helene Nawrocki, R.N., M.S.N., CNA
Exec. Vice-President, Center for Nursing Excellence, Newtown, PA.

"WARNING: If you're completely content with your life and profession, don't read this book! But - if you'd like to break through to higher levels of understanding, performance and healing, *THE NIGHTINGALE CONSPIRACY* can help you get there. This book is rich with insight and wisdom about the soul of nursing..."
Barbara Dossey, R.N., M.S., F.A.A.N.
Director, Holistic Nursing Consultants, Santa Fe, New Mexico
Author: *Critical Care Nursing: Body-Mind-Spirit; Cardiovascular Nursing: Holistic Practice; Holistic Nursing: A Handbook for Practice*

"At long last, nurses are awakening to their true destiny as healers! *THE NIGHTINGALE CONSPIRACY* is significant and timely, as it challenges nurses to claim their power within Healing Health Care. Nurses are in the process of healing themselves in

order to be facilitators of health and healing for others. *THE NIGHTINGALE CONSPIRACY* inspires nurses to unite and look beyond to a new day in the nursing profession. The numbers of nurses conspiring are growing as a result of this heart-centered book!"
Charlotte McGuire, R.N., M.A.
Founder - American Holistic Nurses Association.

"The greatest danger to your health is to give away responsibility for it. This beautifully-told personal story will bring life and love back into the nursing profession as it helps both nurses and the rest of us (including physicians) take back the personal responsibility for our lives."
Gladys Taylor McGarey, M.D.
Past President of the American Holistic Medical Association.

"This revolutionary book is a must for all nurses, physicians, allied health professionals, and health care administrators - those supportive, curious, and concerned about the future of health care and the promise which nursing holds."
Heather Kussman, R.N.C., M.P.A.
Nursing Education Instructor, V.A. Medical Center, San Francisco, CA

"Karilee's strong, loving, and spiritual words represent a professional approach to the problems in a troubled system, offering a challenge for nurses, consumers, and the entire health care institution. She appeals to the heart as well as the intellect, encouraging caregivers to listen to their intuition; to 'nurse healthcare back to health'."
Caryn Summers, R.N.
Author of *Circle of Health and Caregiver, Caretaker: From Dysfunctional to Authentic Service in Nursing.*

the NIGHTINGALE CONSPIRACY

Nursing Comes to Power in the 21st-Century

Karilee Halo Shames, R.N., Ph.D.

Enlightenment Press
1993

2-05

ISBN: 1-884079-15-6

Printed in the United States of America

Cover Design: Gaelyn & Bram Larrick, Lightbourne Images, Kelseyville, CA.

Cover Photo Credit: Morgan Cowin - Photographer, San Rafael, CA.

Selections from *Principle-Centered Leadership,*

COPYRIGHT © 1990, 1991 by Stephen R. Covey.

Reprinted by permission of Simon and Schuster, Inc.

First Edition Published by
Power Publications
56 McArthur Avenue
Staten Island, New York 10312

Revised Second Edition Published by
Enlightenment Press
Healthcare Management Innovations
484 Bloomfield Avenue
Montclair, NJ 07042

9 8 7 6 5 4 3 2 1

In Gratitude...

Any work of art is never accomplished alone. She who gives it birth is merely a channel for Divine Inspiration. This project is the result of a Grand Conspiracy. I feel blessed for my role, with my Guides, Teachers, Higher Power, Family & dear Friends.

I dedicate The Nightingale Conspiracy to Florence Nightingale, whose determination and vision once inspired medicine to be hygienic. May her memory serve as we make it more humane!

Special gratitude to those teachers who shined their light on my path: *Dr. Gladys McGarey, Blossom Bakerman, Darlene Hall, Delores MacManama, Dr. Lisa Robinson, Brig. General Clara Adams Ender, for your faith in me and my dreams.*

Gratitude to my Family of Origin: *Gloria Deutsch Ingraham, for giving me life, and for showing me the tremendous power of woman. I carry the torch of passion out into the world thanks to you! I love you, Mom.*

I. J. Feibus, my Dad, for inspiring me to use my marvelous brain. I hope you know what a great influence you've been!

Sam Feibus, my youngest brother, who taught me of children and will always be near in my heart, and for Gary, Terri, and Ron...

Fanny Feibus & Mae Pearl (Deutsch), my sagacious grandmothers, who gave pearls of wisdom & models of female strength.

Cuz'n Sher, lifelong favorite friend, always there for me. You will forever be a beautiful goddess in my heart. Te adoro siempre...

And to my Present, Chosen Family:
Heartfelt Appreciation to the sacred sisterhood of the American Holistic Nurses Association.

My inspiring AHNA Mentors: Charlotte McGuire, Barbie Dossey, Dorothea Hover, Lynn Keegan, Janet Mentgen, Veda Andrus, Jane Lunt, Peggy Wolfe.

ClarityMae Weber, my nurse empowerment partner and Friend. May our joining be blessed, fruitful beyond our wildest dreams.

Wendy, Carol, Beth, Janne, Raven... my local sisters, who share in the miracles of my daily existence, and to all my AHNA sisters who share their love and light for healthy evolution.

Other Delightful Nurse Conspirators:
Heather Kussman (Guardian Angel) of the VA Education Dept.
David Norris, Founder of National Nurses in Business Association
Merrily (dearest sister & lifelong friend) for birthing my babies so
wonderfully, & for laughing at my weaknesses and honoring my
strengths... for your model of courage and intuition.
Caryn Summers, for your powerful role and gracious support.
Helene Nawrocki and Sandra Crandall...Creators of the Center
for Nursing Excellence...

Thanks to Other Special Friends Along the Path:
Kerry Gardner (Whatever-Your-Name-is-Now), Dianne Duchesne,
Claudia D., & Marta, Denny Ferry, Sylvia (Swann) Vaughn, Loi
Eberle, Arlean Jenks - all of you have helped my growth.
"Gailee", a sister healer and loving friend.
Dhyanis, for awakening my deepest dream to be a dancer.
Gaelyn & Bram Larrick, who have done a magnificent job
creating this cover, and in the process have become my friends.
Bev & John Zeiss, whose vision, expertise, & support have enabled
this book to live on.
Kathy Butler, whose wonderful support will help the conspiracy to grow...

And to My Present Family - Deepest Appreciation for your
daily support in my life:
Rich, my beloved Life Partner & Friend - your strength, vision,
and faith have continually supported my work and growth. I am
deeply honored to walk alongside you on the Great Red Road...
with our delightful children/teachers:
Shauna-Lani Rainbow, lovely, wise firstborn.
Georjana Grace Sunrise ("GiGi"), healing middle child.
Gabriel Benjamin StarDancer, precious son, who teaches us
through his magic.

Disclaimer

With the exception of Loi and Rob Eberle, Richard Shames, Merrily, Dr. Gladys McGarey, and the authors and speakers referenced, the names of all other persons appearing in this work have been changed, and any reference to any persons living or deceased is purely coincidental.

The author gratefully acknowledges permission to reprint excerpts from the following previously published material:

The Aquarian Conspiracy, by Marilyn Ferguson. 1980, J.P. Tarcher/Putman Publishing Group

Backlash, by Susan Faludi. 1991, Crown Publishers

Principle-Centered Leadership, by Stephen Covey. 1990, Summit Books/Simon & Schuster

Think & Grow Rich, by Napoleon Hill. 1960, Ballantine Books/ Napoleon Hill Foundation

Nurses: The Human Touch, by Michael Brown, R.N. 1992, Ballantine Books/Random House

The Prophet, by Kahlil Gibran. 1923, Alfred A. Knopf/Random House

Holistic Nursing, by Dossey, Keegan, Guzzetta, & Kolkmeier. 1988, Aspen Publishers

I'm Dying to Take Care of You, by Candace Snow & David Willard R.N. 1989, A/D Communications, Health Communications

Caregiver, Caretaker, by Caryn Summers, RN. 1992, Commune-A-Key Publishing

How to Choose and Use Your Doctor, by Marvin Belsky MD and Leonard Gross. 1975, Arbor House/Simon & Schuster

The author is also grateful for the information provided in the following supportive works:

Witches, Midwives & Nurses, by Ehrenreich and English. 1973, Feminist Press

"Cassandra", Florence Nightingale, introduction by Myra Stark. 1979, Feminist Press

Nursing: The Finest Art, by M. Patricia Donahue. 1985, C.V. Mosby Co.

Karilee Shames, R.N., Ph.D. offers motivational and
educational seminars for nurses, women, and health care
consumers on a variety of topics related to health, holistic care,
and empowerment issues. She is also available for private
consultation. For a schedule of upcoming seminars or retreats, or
if you are interested in bringing one to your area, please write to
her at:

P.O. Box 2398
Mill Valley, Ca 94942
(415) 388-NEWS

To All Nurses Everywhere - May you all be blessed with Divine Wisdom & Grace, that you may be shown the path to your truest heart, and granted all the support you need to follow it. *May every one of you occupy your perfect role in*

The Nightingale Conspiracy...

The Nightingale Conspiracy

WANTED

POWERFUL NURSES TO LEAD
A HEALTH CARE REVOLUTION

Are you a strong nurse who has been accused of 'speaking out'?

Have you always wanted to work with your hands and heart connected, but found that you must put on a mask and pretend to be other than a healer to do your nursing work?

Are You Ready For A Change?

THE NIGHTINGALE CONSPIRACY is looking for a team of courageous, visionary nurses who are willing to use their hands, hearts, minds, spirits, and strength to create a new model of nursing, one which supports more humane care and consumer empowerment.

Benefits include enhanced self-esteem, relief from burnout, rejuvenation, a deep sense of job satisfaction, and a powerful support network in which to grow and be nourished.

Apply today.

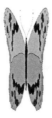

INTRODUCTION

Once, long ago, there was a goddess named Hygeia. She taught that people could remain well if they lived according to reason and moderation. Hygeia symbolized what is known as the feminine principle of health care.

As time passed, Hygeia's popularity gave way to that of Aesculapius, the first physician. He stood for the masculine principle in health care, by battling disease as if it were an unprovoked attack by a hostile enemy.

The myths of Hygeia and Aesculapius illustrate the polarity between two opposite viewpoints in medicine. For worshippers of Hygeia, health is the natural order of things, to which every person is entitled if he or she lives wisely. In this light, nursing's main function (as the professional embodiment of the feminine principle) is to discover and teach the natural laws which will continually provide for a healthy mind in a healthy body.

In today's medical world, excess faith in the battle ethic of

Aesculapius has overshadowed the importance of Hygeia's common-sense wisdom. For a healthier balance, medicine must embrace more of the natural health principles, for only then will we truly enjoy more freedom from dis-ease.

It is my goal to have the hospitals work better and feel healthier for every person, especially the nurses. So often, individual needs are lost in large institutions, and sometimes entire groups are overpowered. Nursing has been one such group.

As nurses, we must begin to appreciate and care for ourselves. Nursing is an art, a unique art, and a science as well. Though we've been taught the scientific principles and methods, many of us wish to express our true nature through a more humane and artistic application of that science. As medicine has become more enmeshed with machinery, the gentle balancing touch of nursing is needed *now more than ever*.

Many nurses entered their training with a vision to inspire and teach people to heal, yet somehow we are seen today as physician's assistants at best, and more often as hospital 'maids' - room service that comes with the bed. There are few avenues open for us to draw salaries commensurate with our years of training and education.

Many of us receiving the highest wages have often traded in the option to use our hands and hearts to become high-tech machine watchers, or managers commissioned to keep a disgruntled group of undernourished and overwhelmed staff nurses in line.

Today's nurses are challenged in many arenas. Government policies and insurance companies now dictate the parameters of health care. These policies affect treatment modalities, a patient's length of stay, and assign limits to care, without considering the

2

individual or the severity of his condition. Therefore, nurses are caring for sicker patients who are often discharged before they are fully able to care for themselves.

Additional financial constraints force health care facilities and agencies to stretch their staff, causing nurses to care for more and sicker patients than ever before. Hospital staffing patterns have not changed significantly to meet the demands of a patient load requiring such intensive care.

Since 97 percent of nurses are women, nursing could truly be the embodiment of the feminine principle in healing (caring, with hands on and hearts open). Instead, we seem to be entangled in all the problems that both doctors *and* professional women face. Not only are our salaries a fraction of what these professionals command, but we also face many problems unique to nursing as well.

Our plight can look bleak, and I could further elaborate on the problems. *I would rather, however, be involved with creating solutions.* As a professional who has travelled as far up on the ladder as she cares to go in the existing hierarchy, as a holistic nurse, and as a writer and counselor who has worked with thousands of nurses, I can speak for one large subgroup of my chosen profession, those who wish to return more to the true roots of a long-lost art, and *put more CARING into CURING!*

During medicine's last great revolution, Florence Nightingale provided 'caring' by defining lifesaving hygienic measures. In the wartime of the mid-1800's, this was urgently needed, and it resulted in nursing being upgraded into a profession. Her contributions produced a quantum leap in British hospital care. Her influence and changes quickly spread around the world, and she is one of the most well-known and respected women of her time.

Currently, a new revolution is needed. There are several missing ingredients necessary to create a true 'health care' system. Initially, the present medical-industrial complex (doctors, hospital corporations, pharmaceutical companies) needs to be balanced and tempered with more humanistic values. The major third party payors (government and private insurance companies) need to see the inherent wisdom in hiring and promoting nurses as health educators and preventive specialists.

The second missing ingredient is *informed consumer involvement.* To help achieve this goal, nursing must immediately enhance its public image, and command more respect in the system. As we improve our self-image and well-being, we can teach health care consumers about these benefits, thus inspiring their empowerment.

The final major ingredient is assertive nursing leadership. To comprehend the grand mission of nursing, let us now consider the concept of 'conspiracy'. Imagine, just for now, that there exists an order in the world that preordains our movement. In other words, consider that our lives are not made of random, haphazard motions, but rather that we have each been called to be here, on this planet, at this time, in our own special way. You were selected to do what you do best - whatever that may be, and likewise, I have been asked to come to 'planet Earth' to offer my very special contributions.

This might be considered, in a positive sense, to be a conspiracy - much as was introduced in the powerful book *The Aquarian Conspiracy* by Marilyn Ferguson in 1980.

'Conspiracy', in the sense intended in this book, means 'to breathe with, or breathe together'. The breath is the force of life, for

as we exchange breath with other living forms, we are nourished. Similarly, as we each breathe in together, our 'spirits' are nourished, and we form a single entity - a collection of beings working together and sharing the force of life. The spirit is considered to be the seat of the soul, where our essence resides.

Breathing together is, when we think about it, big medicine! Conspiring is a way of sharing our common dreams and visions. *Every nurse must begin the personal and professional journey towards feeling whole, in order to become part of a powerful solution together. Every nurse brings special gifts to her work, and is a crucial part of the whole. We are all needed to make it happen.*

This book is intended, through intimate sharing and factual information, to inspire you to strengthen yourself, and to join forces with other nurses, that together we can 'conspire' to creatively solve 'the nursing problem'.

You are urgently needed to take your proper role; to help usher nursing into the 21st-century with a renewed sense of dignity and purpose. . . to then create a healthy revolution in health care. . .

The Nightingale Conspiracy.

PART I

TRUE NURSING

WHAT IS IT, REALLY?

THE HEART OF NURSING
ANCIENT, FEMINIST,
AND MODERN VIEW

Dusk arrives without warning in the small mountain village, casting a beautiful reddish glow onto its people. Tired from their labors, they shuffle slowly into clay dwellings which offer simple shelter from the rains and cold of night. Smoke fills the air, as families gather to share food.

Around the fires, fathers proudly present meat to their offspring, reward of their successful hunt. Young and old alike devour the food, having heard the tales of the warriors' brave ventures into the wilderness. Tonight, the men dance their hunting dance, sharing the story of their catch with those too young or old to join their work.

The mood is joyful, one of celebration for the villagers. In the distance, however, far from the noisy gathering, two people hover to-

gether inside a small hut. Meeting the darkness with silence, they alone do not partake in the evening's festivities. The young girl ministers to her grandmother, who has long been the keeper of herbal knowledge. For many winters, the ancient woman quietly prepared the concoctions with which her people have fought off evil spirits and death.

Tonight though, the older woman faces her own darkness, guided by the gentle loving hand of her granddaughter. The girl bends over her, moistening the leaves upon her forehead with some carefully-brewed potion, as she has watched her grandmother do for many others. The woman speaks in a strange tongue, perhaps visiting a land far away where the ancestors dwell.

As dusk gives way to darkness, the young girl has no thoughts of her own hunger or tiredness, only of the woman with whom she has apprenticed for many moons to prepare herself for her eventual role as caregiver. Now, holding the hand of the dying woman, she wonders if she is yet fully prepared.

Her fear quickly gives way to a stronger power, the knowledge that all things come to pass in their own season, and that as life shows the way, so must we follow the path of our truest heart. The young girl feels the courage of the lion, her totem, and breathes its power onto her healing hands. She relaxes through slow, deep breathing, growing into a peaceful awareness that her time has come. Now she must trust herself to carry on the work of wisdom and compassion, as did her ancestors, the sacred work of ministering to those in need.

The Birth of the Nurse

Who is this young woman, preparing herself for a life of service to those in her community? What is this work that she does with such devotion - her special calling? Does she live in today's world, or is she merely a forgotten memory from a far distant era?

This young girl, keeper of healing wisdom, is the ancient relative of a currently dying breed. She lived long ago, passing her skills on to her daughters and granddaughters, who in turn shared knowledge with their offspring. She lives today in the hearts of several million women in the United States alone, and many more worldwide: women who have heard the call in their youth, as well as women who have been called in their later years to care for community members.

Yet amidst these vast numbers, she is an endangered species, hovering on the edge of annihilation. In earlier times, she was revered for innate responsiveness and dedication. Now, she spends much valuable energy in efforts to validate her contributions to society, to be heard, listened to, and honored. Though she has spent years pursuing formal education, the public still remains confused about her unique abilities, and skeptical of her sometimes seemingly simplistic maneuvers.

She now combines her innate, right-brain wisdom with the left-brain sciences so trusted in today's world, yet still her work is feared and misunderstood. This attitudinal deficit, so prevalent in her culture, undermines her contributions, creating a negative spiral, a deep abyss of darkness and imbalance. Who is this woman, often born and bred of healing stock, who has successfully passed through a dark period where she was burned as evil, and now seeks again to arise of

11

the ashes and create balance in an unbalanced world?

She is the nurse; 'nurturer', caretaker of the body and spirit. She has descended from a long line of women in healing, adding the caring to curing; the gentle touch to balance aggressive scientific interventions.

It is said that at one time the healing work was accomplished by the shaman in the community, the physician-priest. His job was to tend to the physical and spiritual needs of the sick. At some point, there arose a need to separate these tasks, so that one healer was designated to care for the diseased or injured parts of a person in a crisis, while another was called to minister on-going nurturance to promote healing of body, mind, and spirit. In this division of labor, nursing was born.

Throughout the ages, women have been keepers of the hearth, nursemaids to children and the sick. It was a natural evolution for women to take over the caring after the physician had given his magic to the person. In those earlier times, there seemed to be no judgements about which tasks were more crucial, whose powers more potent. There was, instead, a deeper understanding that life was guided by certain principles, forces which did not vary according to personality or persuasion. There was a firm belief in the natural order of life, and each person was honored according to the contributions he/she was able to offer. The shaman was highly respected for his healing powers, and the women who provided nurturing were like-wise honored for their gifts. The understanding seemed to be that all things worked together for the highest good; that each person held a piece of the puzzle in the great mystery of life.

Today, our society seems to have forgotten that each person is blessed with her own special magic, and that we can honor ourselves and each other for the special gifts we all bring. Possibly, there is no group that so suffers from this omission as the nurse, for she has lost her way, and there has been no one to guide her. In trying to fit into the 'scientific', 'professional' model, she has lost her deepest soul.

A Brief 'Herstory' of Modern Nursing

Especially during the past few decades, nursing has undergone major challenges. Prior to 1910, women had a certain amount of freedom to practice their special healing arts. Midwifery flourished, and the work of women was often done by women, for women. There was a great deal of respect given to the instinctual nursing abilities of women as we cared for one another in the sanctuaries of our homes and villages. The wisdom passed down from one generation to the next was powerful medicine, one of its most potent ingredients being the belief of the people. It was a 'people's medicine'.

In the early 1800's, midwives, folk healers, and other practitioners dominated the medical scene. According to Ehrenreich and English in their popular underground pamphlet "Witches, Midwives and Nurses",[1] beginning in the late 19th-century the American public gradually granted the medical profession a monopoly of the healing arts as part of a long era of class and gender struggles. The folk healers used simple, non-invasive herbal remedies. The formally trained doctors (with little actual training) became more accepted, even through their 'cures' were often more injurious than the original disease.

In the 1830's and 1840's, the Popular Health Movement was evidence of a general social upheaval, stirred up by feminists and working class people, in an effort to diminish medical elitism. The 'regular' doctors (more highly trained) were highly outnumbered, while new schools arose to create a more moderate brand of doctor. At the same time, the world felt the first stirrings of organized feminism.

Throughout the latter 19th-century, the 'regulars' attacked lay practitioners. Women were forced to choose sides in this enormous class struggle, and those from middle class upbringing often identified more with the 'regulars' than with the immigrants and lay healers. In this stance, middle class women became identified with the emerging male medical profession.

Around the turn of the century, European scientists identified the germ theory of disease, thus expanding medical knowledge and giving the scientifically-elite 'regular' doctors even more credibility. Foundation money began to be granted in large amounts to 'regular' medical institutions. Johns Hopkins Medical School became the standard by which all medical training was measured, and the Carnegie Corporation sent Abraham Flexner on a national tour to evaluate existing medical schools.

In 1910, the famous "Flexner Report"[2] was published, banishing the 'uneducated' from the realms of healing. The poorer smaller schools, especially those for blacks and women, were discounted. Since the 'elite' universities did not provide education for females, most women were immediately forbidden from tending to the sick, under the guise of concern for public safety.

While there can be no doubt that some individuals of integrity were indeed attempting to protect the masses from 'quackery', it was also known that most males felt threatened by the women's healing powers, and had conspired for several generations to eliminate this feminine competition (dating back to the pervasive witch hunts - and

14

before).

In 1910, 50% of all babies were delivered by midwives. The emerging obstetrical specialty felt highly threatened, especially since their 'teaching cases' were from the lower classes, who patronized the midwives. Even though a study at John Hopkins demonstrated that physicians then were less competent than the midwives, the obstetricians launched a major attack against midwives, virtually eliminating their work.

Nursing's Special Challenge Today

In our sophisticated society, we insist upon scientific proof before we allow medicinals and treatments to be offered, yet how effective are we at truly healing the diseases of our times? Western medicine has demanded that consumers think as the medical-pharmaceutical industry dictates, stripping from those who are ill the right to choose their own healing journey, the quality of their life and death experiences. It is always a major omission to neglect the belief systems of the individuals involved.

In ignoring the obvious power of the 'placebo' effect, and the patient's cultural and religious milieu, we have been steamrolled into accepting a highly invasive, overly technological medical system. As consumers become disempowered and separated from the community's healing potential, they find themselves painfully isolated. What they might find most beneficial is instead to be immersed in the comfort and security of their home surroundings, far away from the sterility of megalithic institutions.

In keeping out the 'germs', we have also taken away much of

our patients' support systems. In the insensitive application of advanced technology, we have stripped away their sense of efficacy, replacing it with our need to dominate and dictate according to our belief systems.

According to Deepok Chopra,[3] an Indian physician who was trained in our country, we further disempower consumers through what he calls the 'nacebo effect'. This phenomenon, as distinguished from the familiar 'placebo effect', occurs when doctors authoritatively convince patients that they are doing poorly.

An everyday example of this occurred years ago when I found a small lump on my thyroid, and the internist immediately sent me to the nearest major medical center for extensive and expensive testing. After many hundreds of dollars of workup, he said he wanted to biopsy it to be sure it wasn't cancer.

I come from a long line of women with autoimmune thyroid disorder, which often presents with an irregular, lumpy gland. The constant presumption that "it could be cancer" began to weigh very heavily on my psyche, and I became quite ill from the combination of immense fear coupled with the added stress of many hours spent with costly and scary machinery, and undue financial burden. The combination of stress and fear was making me sick! I chose, instead, to use homeopathy initially, and later a program of thyroid replacement therapy. Today, I continue on this program, with bounding energy.

Consider what often occurs when a doctor tells a patient that he has only two months left to live. The patient's subconscious mind incorporates this negative programming into his belief system, inspiring the 'good patient' to be compliant, and die within two months.

Dr. Chopra found himself wondering if doctors were correct in

16

their assessment, or whether they were creating the situation by planting negative thoughts in their patients' minds. Since current research has demonstrated the incredible power of the human mind to create our realities according to our belief system, it seems possible that doctors, in making negative suggestions, are actually promoting the acceleration of the patient's demise. Isn't it also possible that, as nurses we have stood witness to this process, and through our nonassertive behavior, have actually participated in negative programming?

What then could be the true role of nursing in our highly-scientific society? Is there still a place for us, a way we can share our special strengths and skills? Are we a dying breed, or merely going through the process of transformation, and experiencing a rebirth?

~   ~   ~   ~   ~

In 1977, another nurse and I joined forces to create an organization called Nurses in Transition. Our dream was to have a chance to support the hundreds, and thousands, of nurses out there who were feeling confused, angry, and ready for a change. At first, our visions matched.

Ten years later, though, after hundreds of support group meetings and weekend workshops, she felt the group had served its purpose, and was no longer needed. I disagreed. She felt that nursing was like a big dinosaur, on the edge of extinction. She thought it ought to be killed and put out of its misery. I totally disagreed.

I thought then, and continue to believe today, that nursing is going through the painful and exhilarating process of rebirth. I see thousands of nurses, in different fields, and different parts of the country, who want it to be different. They want to use their hands

17

and hearts for healing; they want to be healed; and they want to be able to model empowerment for other nurses and for health care consumers.

Nursing's Role in the Emerging Paradigm

In *Nurses: The Human Touch*,[4] Michael Brown, RN, ends by quoting a nursing instructor who perceives a problem for nurses that goes beyond the health care system to the very social agenda of the nation.

> "Quite simply, it is difficult to demand and then receive respect for doing something that society itself takes for granted . . . like motherhood . . . the greatest demand now and for the foreseeable future will be the compassionate care of the sick and dying, which is exactly how nursing got started."[5]

This instructor seems to be alluding to one of nursing's inherent ironies. Despite the myriad technological advances we have witnessed in this last century, she feels that nursing will be in demand at the turn of the century in precisely the same way that it was needed as the century began, in caring for those dying of chronic and infectious diseases. The AIDS epidemic has been a reminder that technology cannot solve every medical challenge, and that in the end, what people continue to need is good loving care.

On the other hand, according to Martha Rogers,[6] nursing theologian, nursing does not corner the market on human caring. At the 1992 National Conference of the American Holistic Nurses Association in Hot Springs, Arkansas, Dr. Rogers carefully articulated in her keynote address that nursing is "not solely caring. Nursing is a body of knowledge, and caring is one of the ways that we use that knowledge."

Dr. Rogers points out that all health practitioners care in their own unique way. Chiropractors express their care through specific manipulations, based on their own extensive education. Nutritionists express their care through sharing their knowledge about food and how nutrients support the human frame. Medical doctors have their own body of knowledge, and base their care upon these theories.

Nurses, according to Dr. Rogers, have a unique body of knowledge, one which lends itself to a heightened understanding of humanity, and which can be used creatively for enhanced well-being. As she sees it, the proper movement for nursing in the 21st-century is toward more non-invasive, whole person therapies. Since each science is identified by its focus, she invites us to see nursing as a science of human beings, based on teachings of Hygeia and Florence Nightingale. Nursing is, and must remain, distinct, an art unto itself, and not to be confused with medicine.

From Rogers' presentations and writings comes the larger vision: our culture has been preparing for hundreds of years for a 'paradigm shift', a new way of thinking and looking at life. Modern science is rooted in the world view of reality, and that world view is about to undergo a major transformation. After thousands of years of looking at the world in a certain way, we are reaching the critical mass for a new way of thinking.

~   ~   ~   ~   ~

Confusion reigns in the health care system today. A troubled economy is creating the need for health care consumers to take more and more responsibility for their treatment. Families are increasingly participating in the care of other family members, and we are gradually returning to a concept of community.

These changes are occurring rapidly, and will continue. Natural disasters, which have been predicted consistently for this transitional time on our planet, are escalating, also insuring the return of a sense of connectedness to one another.

Though these changes may seem frightening to many people, they also have their beneficial aspects, particularly with regard to our human needs for caring and socialization. Technological alienation cannot persist when people are forced by necessity to live together as community members facing life-threatening conditions.

There are some much needed rewards as we face these challenging times. For the last few decades, our technological advances have far surpassed our ability to use them wisely. As nurses, we have certainly been silent witness to this proliferation and its devastation. As a planet, we have been on the brink of annihilation, thanks to our advances in nuclear and germ warfare.

What will save us will be our sense of spiritual connectedness, our reverence for all life forms, and our growing awareness of the need for balance. These changes require the joining of minds of clear-thinking, assertive individuals, ones who place the welfare of the whole above their own personal needs or benefits.

What has been occurring in medicine has been quite different. Insurance companies and the profit-oriented medical/pharmaceutical industry have continued to dictate policy and treatment. Now we recognize the increased need for consumer empowerment.

Empowerment occurs when we feel efficacious, and recognize that we can protect ourselves in any unsafe or unhealthy situation. It comes from knowing that we have the skills, tools, information, and support with which to make healthy changes. It comes as we each personally empower ourselves, then model empowerment so nurses can learn from each other how to be effective and powerful as leaders. These concepts will be discussed in great length in the final chapter of this book, Nurse Empowerment.

Power can be defined as *the ability to influence change.* Now that we nurses realize the urgent need for healthy changes in our medical system, it is imperative that we join forces to create synergy. Now is the time for nursing to rise to its full glory, promoting healing with our hands, hearts and souls aligned.

There is no other profession so perfectly suited to empower people to care for themselves and each other as the nursing profession. We arose out of the need for communities to take care of their members and promote well-being amongst the group, and nursing's domain is still designed to inspire healing.

As we contemplate the needed restructuring of our society, never has there been a time so ripe for supporting the empowerment of professional women healers. Even this brief review of history can remind us that women have been honored as healers at times in the past. Yet never before have we had the opportunity to be highly educated and to practice our special healing arts with the benefit of our advanced knowledge.

Today there are more men joining the ranks of nursing, yet it remains a predominantly female field (97%). It is also women's first attempt at professionalization. Guided (as both males and females) by the feminine principle, which supports the receptive inward heal-

21

ing abilities, modern nursing is a diverse conglomerate of tasks, perhaps encompassing the work of at least twenty known fields.

There are many nurses today working in health-related, non-nursing practices. Some of these people do not consider their work nursing, others clearly do. Nonetheless, as nurses increasingly enter the hallowed halls of law, of technology and engineering, of medicine and insurance, and even as nurses embark upon their journeys as private practitioners in the healing arts, we are re-creating nursing and further recognizing its grandest potential.

As we expand the scope of our work into the gray interface between art and science, between medicine and sociology, between folklore and technology, we are pushing the definition of nursing to create our own science.

Nursing has generally had the advantage of the public's trust. Whereas medicine in this century has aligned itself with a god-like position, great economic interest, and increasing dictatorship policies based on fear and lack of consumer awareness, nursing has worked towards the opposite end. Many nurses are hopeful that physicians will take the example and work more collaboratively with nurses and patients. Whether we like it or not, nursing and medicine are interdependent in today's system.

Nursing, in its clearest endeavor, strives to empower the consumers through providing the skills, tools, information, and support with which to make healthy decisions about life.

In a report issued by the Department of Health & Human Services,[7] the findings of a public group of chosen national leaders speak to the specialness of nursing, and it's enormous societal value:

Nursing is a resource invaluable to the nation's

health . . .

Today, nursing means working in difficult and complex situations. It requires being able to think clearly and professionally. It requires using experience, sensitivity and creativity to make critical and often urgent decisions. Nursing takes leadership, initiative, managerial expertise, and increasingly, advanced education. It is work in which complexity and emotional strain are continually encountered, often leading to job dissatisfaction and career disillusionment . . .

The need for knowledgeable, sophisticated, caring nurses is greater now than any time in the profession's history . . .

. . . the time has come to examine and redefine the role and functions of the nurse. The vital role of nursing in relation to American health care priorities must be articulated. A full and ongoing dialogue between nursing and its public is crucially important to the renegotiation of the contract between nursing and society. This is the essential task facing nursing and society over the next decade. (emphasis added)

Nursing's Specialness

To truly understand the grand mission of nursing, we now have to consider the ways in which our collective, nonassertive, codependent tendencies might have further contributed to the problem, instead of the solutions. If we were to view the patient as more than just a sick body (which already distinguishes us from the medical model), we would allow ourselves to recall the deep spiritual values out of which nursing was born. We would remember that the early nurses were the healers in the communities, often the devoted sisters of religious orders, and that the early nurse cared for the body, mind, and spirit of the ailing person.

Perhaps we have also gotten side-tracked by our affiliation with devoted religious caregivers. We have come to see ourselves as the modern caretakers of the human soul and spirit, yet in today's world we have no support systems such as the nurse-nuns had in previous times. We have been attempting to follow in their footsteps, demurely and docilely caring for our patients, yet living with enormous pressures that they did not have to face.

Nurses today are frequently mothers, many are single parents, who have rent and bills to pay that nurses in the days gone by did not have. According to Maslow's hierarchy of needs,[8] we must first assert ourselves in assuring that our basic needs are met if we are ever to reach our loftier goals. To truly nurse in the most glorious manner, we must take the ideals that are still near and dear to our hearts and modify them according to our abilities, setting appropriate boundaries to maintain our own health and well-being. We are modern nurses, and we must adapt.

Florence Nightingale was the 'Lady with the Lamp', the one who tenderly walked through the Crimean battlefields shining light on the wounded, touching them briefly in the dark hours of the soul, when they struggled between life and death. Often it was her touch that moved something within them, some spark of will that grew into a desire to live, to return home to loved ones, to trust that life had more to offer. Many of these young men remembered that her light awakened their dreams, and for those small moments of inspiration, they offered deep gratitude. That small touch that nursing offers can make all the difference.

Could Western Medicine exist without its nurses? Are we worthy of demanding that our basic needs be met and commanding great respect in the medical system? I believe our contributions are invaluable, unique, and absolutely necessary.

In an attempt to alleviate the nursing shortage, the physicians recently tried to create a new category of health care worker, the 'Registered Care Technician'. To me, it seems a move similar to the creation of the more advanced category of 'Physicians Assistant'.

These people ultimately have the potential to take over much of the work that nurses have been doing today, and yet I feel strongly that medicine could never exist without the gentle touch of nursing, without the special form of caring that inspired nursing to be created. In many ways, my instinctive response is that we should let the physicians create as many categories of helpers as they need, all under their jurisdiction, and nursing would thus be freed up to do what we do best, guided by our own innate wisdom and intuition.

The masculine principle (fighting disease as if it were an enemy) must always be balanced with the feminine principle (allowing the disease process to teach us about the ways in which we have been trying to live outside the laws of nature). They go together quite nicely, but one will never replace the other. In the ancient Eastern concept of Yin/Yang, or male/female, it is known that life seeks balance. In our ultra-masculine medical world, nursing in its truest form is now needed much as a thirsty plant desperately craves water.

In fact, to many of us nurses, it occurs that our special 'medicine' is exactly the remedy needed to cure our ailing medical system. Strong, powerful nursing guidance could significantly change the direction of runaway medical treatment... skyrocketing costs (dictated in part by the physician lifestyle), iatrogenic illness (physician-caused disease), defensive medicine (painful expensive procedures done to consumers to protect the doctors, and to prevent the lawyers from getting their money). All these are battles currently being played out with government and insurance monies, which ultimately come from the consumers of health care. And though the nurses' salaries remain a mere fraction of these other male-orientated professions, our worth is immeasurable.

From Ancient China came a belief, "The Mandate of Heaven", which said that leadership is spiritually obvious, stemming from the will of the people. It seems that every few hundred years in the dynastic cycle there was a major upheaval, in which the rulers were replaced with new ones through the collective joining in the will of the common people. At this time, nursing has the "mandate of heaven". The public still trusts us, and knows that we have their best interests at heart, but we have not demonstrated our strength, cohesiveness, and leadership in a way that inspires them to stand fully behind us. This is the challenge we face today - in order to live fully in our glory.

Summary

As the Secretary's Commission on Nursing discovered, it is now up to us, as nurses, to emerge as powerful leaders in health care. It is our challenge to articulate who we are to a confused public, and to command their support for the mutual goals we share.

As we overcome any sense of victimization, as we recognize fully who we are and what the task is, and as we claim our proper place in society, the balance will be restored. We, as nurses, are entrusted with the care of the consumers on a whole-person level. We are not only here to care for the body, but also the soul and spirit.

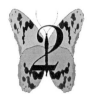

'HERSTORY'
A LOST ART
AND
TARNISHED IMAGE

As we further delve into our story, we can learn more about the ways we have lost contact with nursing's creative potential, thus causing a tarnishing of our image. In doing so, we can release that which no longer serves us as nurses, and recover that which touches our hearts and makes us whole. The journey through the past will inevitably support us in creating a future that is more aligned with who we are as nurses. As we examine our previous experiences, we begin to discover more about the psyche of the nurse.

Who is she? What special gifts does she bring to the world? Where did she lose her way, and why did she allow it to happen? It would promote our collective well-being to answer some of these questions.

In recapturing our initial dreams individually, we can unite them to build something beautiful and more meaningful for ourselves and those we serve. In examining our tarnished image, we learn from our weaknesses to develop our strengths.

The journey to empowerment takes dedication. It requires a willingness to face the darkness, to move through it, and also a desire to live in the light. This concept may seem strange, even foreign, to nurses, as nursing has maintained a victimized consciousness, and a belief that evil things have been done to us. In choosing empowerment, we accept the responsibility to 'face our dragons, and know that they are us'.

Victims tend to attract perpetrators by virtue of their weakened posture and self-image. If nursing's image has been tarnished, we must hold ourselves partly accountable for the damage, and for the restoration. Though this may seem an ominous task, it can readily be accomplished through the synergy we can create by joining together.

Victims believe that all harmful or negative circumstances arise outside of themselves, and that they have no control over the situation. Assuming an empowered posture, we agree to face the shortcomings within us all, including any weaknesses which have contributed to our professional demise. As we begin to shift, and make changes in our behavior and attitudes, we create shifts in the system. Like dominoes, one change results in a change in every other interconnected part. Like the pebble thrown into a pond, ripples go outward into the world whenever we make a 'splash', no matter how small.

In assuming responsibility, we need not blame nor feel worse about ourselves, but rather make the decision to learn what we can from every experience and move on. When similar situations occur again, we can face them with more knowledge and courage, incorporating the necessary changes.

As promoters of healthy change, we are learning to take risks, willing to make mistakes (a new concept for many nurses), and trusting that we will be guided towards a happier, healthier life by these attitudinal changes. When we change how we feel about ourselves, we change the world. When we begin to see ourselves through new eyes, we change our image in the eyes of others.

What is an Image?

An image is a symbol; a representation that stands for something else. Florence Nightingale carried an oil lamp on evening rounds through the battlefields and barracks of the Crimea. This image became crystallized in many minds:

The nurse is a devoted, caring person, tending to the sick and injured amidst the ravages of an often brutal world. She sees what is needed, takes charge, and makes sure the job is done properly, even if that means working late and long hours.

Florence's image continues to inspire us. It lights our fires of faith and desire. We yearn to follow in her footsteps at times, to be seen as brave, to be known as wise. Deep within, we nurses know how powerful and wise we are, for our knowledge springs from an eternal source. We speak of hygiene, and wholeness, yet have felt strangled in our sharing, misunderstood in our caring, uncertain of how to proceed.

"The journey of 1000 miles begins with a single step." Thus teaches China's ancient book of wisdom, the Tao Te Ching. Yes, we're painfully aware of the challenges nurses face, but we also understand that our challenges bring out our strength, and nursing has much that is strong. We have many tools at our disposal for healing, both for ourselves and others. We've learned well to use the scientific method, but we also see the wisdom of turning inside ourselves for solutions. We can encourage others to start seeing us differently, while simultaneously envisioning ourselves whole, seeing ourselves as powerful, creating nursing's new image in our own mind's eye. We are beginning to understand how very powerful that process of revisioning can be.

Nursing has been accused of being schizophrenic - the sinner and the saint, the Madonna and the whore. It is true that nursing has had many faces, and is continually acquiring more. Too much valuable time has been spent reflecting on these differences, however, and not enough on our similarities. Now is the time to heal this omission.

In our attempts to visualize the problem we face, consider that we might use a special tool. If we had a powerful multi-view projector to help bring nursing's various images into focus, we could merge these individual pictures into a hologram, one three-dimensional representation of our profession.

We could all shine our individual lights together in such a way as to radiate one clear image outward. *To clarify our image, we must now synthesize nursing's multidimensional nature into one focused picture.* Once we have achieved this ability, once we grasp the awareness that nursing in its many faces can have one common image, then we can begin to radiate that image outward. We can each more easily merge our individual effort with that of the whole. In addition, those outside the profession can use the image to feel closer and more supportive of nurses. This ability helps to demonstrate why positive images are so powerful.

An 'image' can be a likeness, or representation. It can be an actual or mental picture drawn by the fancy, a type, as in 'she is the image of devotion'. After considering the image of Florence Nightingale, let us now focus on another similar image - the Statue of Liberty - standing in New York Harbor. She, too, holds a light, shining it outward to meet the darkness. What is the difference in these two images? As many nurses have suggested, the statue stands for freedom, the other . . . ? (many nurses have answered 'bondage', further evidence of the need to heal our victimization).

There is something else that is different about these images. One is of a real woman - flesh and blood - who was making her contributions to life. The other is merely the giant metal and mortar form of a woman who never existed. As we seek to create a new image, let us remember that we are *real* people, with a *real* mission, and that we must convey who we are clearly and accurately. We cannot allow ourselves to be distracted by incongruent images, but must go about our work with clarity of purpose and integrity. In this manner, we can contribute to the image of the nurse as healer. How nicely our work and mission coincide; as we heal ourselves, we can be healing our image and those we serve as well.

Thus far, the media is confused, the public is confused, and we have been unclear. It is up to us to restore the balance and clear our own image. Now is the time to consolidate the various faces of nursing into one which we can gladly present to the public we serve.

In attempting to create a new image for nursing's future, my words are directed to the heart of every nursing caregiver, including Student Nurses, Nurses Aides, Licensed Practical Nurses, Associate Degree Nurses, Diploma Nurses, Registered Nurses, Nurse Practitioners, Clinical Specialists, Nurse Midwives, Nursing Educators, and Nursing Administrators. We come in many shapes and sizes, many colors and ages, and in a couple of sexes, yet together we comprise one body - the nursing community of America - and it is together that we will overcome the misrepresentation that has plagued our profession.

Nursing's Image Today: Sexpot, Battle-axe, or Angel of Mercy?

An examination of nursing's current image will shed some light on where we need to go toward creating a new image, towards healing ourselves and our profession. Presently, the image of the nurse is disparate, confused, and oftentimes degrading. The most recent media portrayals seem to continue a tradition of casting the nurse in the role of sexpot, most often with minimal brain power.

Several years ago, as the shortage progressed, there was a series of television talk shows featuring panels of nurses, often irate and defensive about their work dilemmas. Rather than finding sympathetic audiences, we found that the public response was to see the nurse as malevolent, the cause of anguish through willful neglect.

Frequently the commentators attempted to go for our jugular - nursing's sore spot - by pitting the nurses one against the other. Though this has not been difficult to achieve, the result is intended to be sensational, rather than restorative. The real heart issues often take a back seat to nursing's incongruities. The frustrated public does not know where to turn to vent its anger and fear. When nurses have gone public to share their views, they have frequently found a less-than-sympathetic audience. Why does this occur?

I have my own ideas about this phenomenon. First, I think the public requires massive educational efforts in order to begin to understand the complex power structure and hierarchy of the hospital corporations. Since the nurse is the one who is there, present, and emotionally as well as physically available, she is often the one to take the blame. It is similar to how we may feel when we come home from a difficult day at work, and a loving spouse or family member is there. All it may take is the slightest provocation for us to let go of our anger and blow off steam. It happens because they're there, and they care, and we need to do something with the seething frustration inside. Often rage comes out inappropriately, frequently at someone we care about and trust.

Perhaps it is similar in the hospitals. When nurses had more time, we used to love to sit at the bedside and talk to the patient and his family, listen to their fears, soothe their aching hearts, and even give the much-needed backrub.

Now, especially with the budget cuts and short staffing, we consider ourselves lucky if we can find the time to point out the patient's room to anxious family members. So, they are scared, and frustrated, and angry.

And if we're honest about it, so are we. We are supposed to be there to help them, and we want to, but who is helping us? Perhaps one solution would be for the hospital corporations to supply customer relations personnel to handle administrative shortcomings, leaving the nurses to do more of our precious work with the patients.

It is also time for us to solicit more cooperation and support from our administrators, to establish some healthy nursing boundaries, and learn to recognize when the problem is *theirs.*

Our problem is that we feel harassed and angry, and have had no place to go with it. One immediate solution is to create and promote more support groups, both within and outside of institutions, where we can share our fears and visions.

What are some other images of nursing? Besides being seen as understaffed and overworked, many professionals have branded us "typically female, unable to agree on anything". They have expressed their frustration with nursing's internal strife and lack of professional cohesion.

Nursing, with its curious educational structure, seems to have been plagued with a non-cooperative spirit. This may be either a reflection or a result of 'the bleeding in our souls' - an occupational hazard. Nurses have felt beaten down, victimized, unsupported, and demoralized. How will we choose to resolve this crisis?

Major changes face us today. Our recent image has indeed been confusing. We have maintained a low profile, a rather strange form of professional privacy, coming to the public's attention (ironically) only when there are not enough of us.

We can no longer quietly go about our work. Now we *must* come to the public's attention, like the Statue of Liberty, shining our beacons of light outward so that everyone can find the way home to their hearts.

History teaches us from our mistakes. We are now beginning to see that we made some serious errors for which we have paid dearly. We were warned by nursing leaders of the last century of the perils of turning over our power, and we did not heed their warning. Now we face a most difficult challenge - that of reclaiming our strength.

In order to better understand the challenges nursing faces today, let us briefly highlight some turning points in our history. A beautiful tribute to the nursing profession, a book called *Nursing: The Finest Art*,[9] was created by M. Patricia Donahue, Ph.D., R.N. In this work of art, Dr. Donahue illuminates much of our history through pictures and descriptive passages.

Our Roots: The Historical Perspective

As we become more aware of our heritage, we begin to see how nursing itself unwittingly contributed to the present day confusion. Though painful at times, this can be an uplifting experience.

According to Donahue, nursing has always been plagued by frustration, ignorance, and confusion. Interestingly, it has also served to mirror both the humanitarian aspects of society at a given time, and also its treatment of women. Human history is certainly marked with times of despair, and during these times nursing has faced greater challenges as well. Though nursing care has always been a necessity in one form or another, our own inability to value our worth has diminished our contributions.

As with the women's movement, much of our value has not been recorded, since men were generally the only ones trained to record. We can observe that early nursing provided the beginnings of community service, and has always had religious connections.

Initially, women were caregivers in the home. The nurturing, nourishing role was something that women were expected to perform for their immediate and extended family. As time went on, the needs grew, families changed in their shape, and nursing skills were used for other people, first extending out to tribe members, and eventually the community at large.

Very early history shows us that the caregivers were occasionally men, sometimes of special religious orders, who provided nurturing to people during times of illness. Some of these men lived in monasteries and dedicated their lives to service, feeling this was their calling. During the Crusades, special groups of knights were created to minister to the sick and injured.

In the Middle Ages, the idea of the hospital was born. More people were then concentrated in one location. As populations grew, so did the concept of nursing and caring for community members. The Renaissance brought renewed interest in the arts and sciences. Along with that came more medical research, enhancing the quality of care available. During the Reformation, as Christianity divided into many sects, there was a shortage of nurses. This period, from 1550 to 1850 has been referred to as 'Nursing's Dark Period'.

Prior to this, the caretakers felt their work was a special calling, and were usually either monks or nuns. When Catholicism began to split into many subgroups, a huge void in nursing developed, as the Catholic nuns were removed from hospital caretaking. The quality of people who were then attracted to nursing were just the opposite of the nuns, with their deep sense of dedication. In fact, in England, women who were serving jail sentences for being misfits were given an opportunity to serve out their jail sentence by working as nurses! Other nurses were pulled from the ranks of alcoholics, lower-class women, and those who had no families or money. No longer was nursing a noble profession, but instead it became a very difficult

38

experience. (I wonder if it was during this time that our profession developed some of its schizophrenic image?)

During the Age of Revolution, great advances occurred in society. It was during this time that Florence Nightingale was invited to support the British soldiers during the Crimean War. War times have always seen increases in the nursing population, since more people require nursing care. During each of the wars involving the U.S., our government deemed it necessary to allocate special funding to train additional nurses.

I was sent through a baccalaureate program during the Viet Nam war as an Army nurse! Though I'm thankful to Uncle Sam, I've often wondered if our wars would be as frequent or as lengthy if nurses weren't so available to pick up the pieces and put the boys together so they can go back and fight. Even Florence Nightingale, in her essay called "Cassandra",[10] wrote about her moral concerns and questionable relationship with and assistance to the British Army.

Up until the Victorian era, however, there was no official training for nurses. Almost anyone could be a nurse, since there was no quality control. In 1850, Nightingale established the Nightingale Training School for Nurses. Even as she shared and created her vision, she was laughed at and ridiculed, though her nature was to pursue relentlessly. Nurses were not treated then with much respect, particularly by the doctors, and had to work under great duress just to provide their service.

In her book, *Notes on Nursing*,[11] Nightingale shared a vision which was the forerunner of today's holistic health philosophy. She always stressed the importance of treating the whole person, and understood her work to be that of strengthening the person's reserve and constitution. With regard to the future of her profession, she was adamant:

> "No system can endure that does not march. Are we walking to the future, or to the past? Are we progressing or are we stereotyping? We remember that we have scarcely crossed the threshold of uncivilized civilization in nursing. There is still so much to do. Do not let us stereotype mediocrity. We are still on the threshold of nursing. In the future, which I shall not see for I am very old, may a better way be opened. May the methods by which every infant, every human being have the best chance of health, the methods of which every sick person will have the best chance of recovery be learned and practiced. Hospitals are only an intermediate state of civilization, never intended in all events to take in the whole sick population."[12]

With these words, the founder of modern nursing handed over the baton to a new generation. In her time, as she envisioned nursing, she did not feel it was, or needed to be, a profession. To her, nursing was a calling, an inner direction.

Since her time, however, the world has wholeheartedly embraced technology, with nursing becoming much more complicated than she could have imagined. Nursing has faced the challenge of this era unprepared in many ways to meet the demands. Physicians, on the other hand, have been able to capitalize on technological change. They have managed, perhaps unwittingly, to make the public continually more dependent on ever newer and more expensive medical intervention.

It should not be too surprising then, after reviewing the history, to more fully understand the need of organized medicine to control all factions of health care. We should not take it too personally, for indeed it has been an enduring pattern for the 'medical men' to eliminate more and more of their competition. In this light, perhaps it is time to give ourselves hearty congratulations for managing to survive thus far!

Some physicians continue to display open hostility to nurses in the hospital setting, though nurses are currently reporting that the younger medical students in recent times demonstrate more respect. Hopefully, as more and more women enter medicine (which is happening rapidly) and more men choose to enter nursing, the time will approach when we can all overcome the gender stereotypes and incorporate our complimentary skills as team members, guaranteeing the improvement of health care.

To complete nursing history in the present century, as early as 1913, Lydia Hall inspired a holistic model at the Global Center for Nursing and Rehabilitation of the Montefiore Hospital in New York. The nurse was, in this setting, the primary caretaker, while medicine and the other arts were considered ancillary.

Other hospital attempts to try and reproduce this model were frustrating due to insufficient staffing, too much emphasis on efficiency, and lack of respect for patient orientation. Still, nursing had shown that it could be done, planting seeds for an eventual time when nursing in its original powerful form could rise again.

Another major influence on nursing at this time was World War I. Prior to this, the majority of the nurses were practicing outside the hospital, enjoying high prestige as public health nurses in the community. The war time economy and patriotic appeal brought most nurses into the hospital situation, where we seem to have gotten stuck, despite the crying need to bring nurses back into community care, and despite our crying need to be autonomous.

Another interesting fact is that at this time, almost half of the nurses working in hospitals were private duty nurses - hired by families - not hospital employees. In this situation, they commanded much more respect and could truly be the patient's advocate.

Another significant milestone occurred in 1928 with the publication of "Nursing, Patients, and Pocketbooks",[13] a report by the Committee on the Grading of Nursing Schools, focusing on the supply and demand of nursing service. This study demonstrated an enormous conflict at that time between nurses and their employers. The service that student nurses were expected to provide as part of their hospital work was often at odds with the school of nursing's objectives.

At the time, training schools were in hospitals, and the hospitals felt that they owned the nurses, hence they got into the habit of using students as cheap labor. With no salaries, the eager students were still able to get a lot of work done. Eventually, it became obvious to the nursing instructors that if nursing was ever to rise above the ranks of where it had been, it needed to be promoted to a higher position.

Now, I ask you, why haven't we come a longer way? More than sixty years later, nurses are still trying to separate from the jurisdiction of hospitals and figure out where nursing belongs!

Another country, our neighbor Canada, has significantly altered the course of American nursing by supplying us with three of our prominent nursing leaders, Isabel Stewart, Lavinia Dock, and Adelaide

Nutting.

Isabel Stewart was very clear about where nursing belonged. She was a prolific writer and worked for many nursing organizations, both national and international. Among her books were *A Short History of Nursing* (1920 - which she wrote with Lavinia Dock) and *The Education of Nurses* (1943). As the years passed, Ms. Stewart expressed concern about the loss of the humanitarian aspects, which had been such a vital force in nursing. Around 1940, she was quoted from a letter to Lillian A. Hudson as saying:

> "I feel very strongly these days that we are failing to develop the social and humanistic side of nursing, the spirit of nursing, as we used to call it, and all that goes to the balancing of the scientific and technical aspects. It would mean a restudy of that whole area dealing with the philosophy and history of nursing and the social sciences, and the strengthening of our cultural roots... I am distressed to realize that we are doing less in the field than we did a few years ago and there seems to be very little interest in it."[14]

Nursing shortages occurred periodically throughout the 20th century. Many nurses stopped practicing to devote time to their family responsibilities, and did not return. Donahue suggests that this may well have been "their answer to an authoritarian and paternalistic system in which they had no participation in planning or decision-making."[15] Many refused to be involved in a system that offered long hours, hard labor, and low pay, all of which undermined their sense of self-esteem and personal power.

(It is noteworthy that we seem to have taken such a silent approach

43

to such a screaming problem. Once again, perhaps if we had used our
voices back then, we would not be fighting the same battles today.)

Lavinia Dock was another very outspoken nurse, who questioned the long-term effects of women's inferior status in health care. A radical feminist, it was her belief that male supremacy in medicine would strongly effect the future of nursing. In the 1930's, she spoke out vehemently against the masculine domination in medicine, which she felt certain would undermine nursing's efforts.

Unfortunately, the nursing leaders of her time ignored her advice, and in the second decade of the century were demoted to non-voting members of the American Hospital Association. They continued to offer support to physicians and administrators (isn't that just like us?), hoping the men in power were interested in helping to solve nursing problems. In this way, physicians and hospital administrators came to be in positions of control over nursing and health care. This same imbalance in health care continues to plague nursing's efforts today.

Another Canadian nurse who made valuable contributions to nursing was Mary Adelaide Nutting. She felt that the nurses needed to be much more involved in creative and critical thinking. It was her vision to see nursing education rise to the university level. As technology increased, nursing became more complex. Nurses needed to learn to identify subtle changes in their patients' condition, learn increasingly complex techniques, increase their ability to interpret laboratory information, and work with newly created drugs with many unknown side effects. In this way, nursing moved more into the realms of doctoring, a journey which has been seen as the downfall of nursing for many.

The Lost Art

The true art of nursing is much more than helping doctors practice medicine. While today there are many nurses who enjoy the challenge of high-level western medicine, many other nurses weep for the loss of their ability to use hands, heart, and head in more natural and traditional ways. For this reason, more and more nurses are feeling drawn to the 'Nightingalean' concepts of holistic health.

Since 1970, holistic nursing has grown stronger and stronger, once again allowing nurses to identify with their role as patient advocate. As more facilities experiment with primary caretaking, natural healing modalities, and collaborative management, nurses once again find themselves in a position to create a healing environment. Many nurses today report using hand-on healing techniques to relax their patients, resulting in a reduction of medications required. Nurses involved in these endeavors are beginning to feel more at home in nursing than they have for a long time.

Isn't there room for all nurses to feel at home in nursing, no matter what our preferences for caring? Can each of us be a valued team member and make our contributions in the way that suits us the best? I certainly think so, and feel that increasing our knowledge about our strong roots and rich heritage will ensure a brighter future.

Co-Dependency: Nursing's Achille's Heel

In order to best imagine how we appear as nurses, we must view nursing in a family context. Recently several well-known authors, including John Bradshaw[16] and Anne Wilson Schaef[17] have expressed deep concern about our national tendency towards addiction.

45

Anne Schaef contends that we are already a nation of addicts. If we consider the many subtle forms of addiction, we can even view the entire medical profession as addicted (to the notion that it is in control of forces which, in fact, can never be harnessed). These beliefs can only be maintained through the use of psychological mechanisms, including denial and repression. To see how this belief is played out, we can consider the health care system as one family group within the larger society.

When medicine is viewed as a family system, doctors are seen as the father, the paternal figurehead. Organizationally, M.D.'s have indeed chosen a 'Big Daddy' style of leadership in which they are the unquestioned authority. They have kept most of the power, in the form of decision-making and financial benefits, for their group. Their commanding presence has intimidated most of the collaborative health workers as well as the patients. As 'captains' of the medical ship, they have freely dictated through what has been routinely accepted as 'Doctor's Orders'.

If the M.D. has been the father, who has been the co-dependent mother in our health care family system? There can be no other answer to this question than 'nurses'. Together, doctors and nurses have lived in big houses (called 'hospitals') with lots of children ('patients'). There is, however, something very unhealthy about this. On closer examination, we can see rampant evidence of dysfunction.

We are not often aware of the problems of the mother or father. In hospitals, as in other dysfunctional families, there are many secrets. Today, one of the biggest of those secrets is beginning to leak out. We are becoming aware that many doctors and nurses are struggling with actual drug addictions. Small wonder! We have easy access and constant exposure to a great selection of pain-altering drugs, and have not received training on changing our own internal chemistry without external drugs, though there is vast evidence that we readily have the power to do this.

We have also lived within the myth of perfection, insisting that we adhere to stringent personal and professional standards, without many healthy outlets available to allow for emotional release or physical relaxation. *(For decades, Dr. Elisabeth Kubler-Ross has been pushing for special rooms in hospitals, where patients and staff can rage or grieve loudly; I have yet to see one).* Perfection, the mask we are expected to don in our professional lives, insists that we become more than human, an untenable task!

These stresses, coupled with immense pressure, constant exposure to society's pain, quarreling with other 'family members' (administration, allied health workers, technicians, etc.), sleep deprivation and interruption, unusual and very extended work hours, and others, have led us to resort to drastic measures to cover up our hurts, our pain, or fear.

Small wonder so many of our ranks have slipped into patterns of drug usage to keep up the charade. For a beautiful description of this problem, I refer you to *Caregiver, Caretaker: from Dysfunctional to Authentic Service in Nursing* by Caryn Summers, RN.[18]

If the doctors have set the oppressive tone for the 'hospital' household, what has been the nurse's role? The nurse seems to have compliantly adapted to the situation, providing a balance by countering the doctor's stern authoritarianism with a soft, 'feminine' response. ("Yes, dear".)

Nurses have become, in addiction jargon, the codependents, or enablers. We are the ones who, by lack of boundary definition and

47

assertiveness, have allowed it to happen. This concept will be further explored in a later chapter.

In this framework, it is easy to see where we nurses took the downward spiral into our present state of dis-ease. We can see the role every person has played in the demise of health care. On a more positive note, however, *this awareness is the first step towards recovery.*

By allowing ourselves to feel beaten down and overpowered by the medical system, we have adopted a victim's stance. We have allowed 'them' to be the authorities on all health care. However, as we move out of the victimized consciousness, we can start to see more clearly why nursing was created in the first place. We are learning to master the process of self-empowerment, so that we can restore ourselves to our rightful position as collaborating professionals.

Nursing's Health Role and Image

Now we can look more closely at the concept of '*health*', in order to refresh ourselves about our true role. Health exists on a continuum from severe illness to high level wellness, with average health in between. According to licensure, medicine is licensed to deal with issues of illness, while nursing is licensed to deal with issues of health:

--Severe Illness---------Average Health------High Level Wellness--

Medicine's Licensure: Nursing's Licensure:

   Authorizes physicians   Authorizes nurses to

    to be 'illness fighters'   be 'health promoters'

In many ways, we nurses have unwittingly become martyrs to an overbearing medical-industrial complex. Its addictive need to have power and control has left us feeling weak and helpless. Moreover, it has created an imbalance (dis-ease) for everyone involved. We have all suffered, doctors included. Now, with increased awareness of the problems, we can begin to pursue healing, first for ourselves, and then for everyone.

Just as the members of Alcoholics Anonymous heal themselves through the twelve step programs, so can nurses begin to cease their codependency. It is time to do it differently; time to rededicate our hospitals into temples of healing. Nurses desperately need to support each other through this delicate restoration.

Is Nursing viable? Is it a female species, destined to devour itself (like the mythical Uroburos, a tail-eating monster), going in circles and eating itself alive? Not only have we been devouring ourselves through lack of support, but we have also been accused of 'eating our young', chewing up and spitting out our brave new graduates, demoralizing them from the start.

Do we possess the internal fortitude to recognize our limitations, to see how our terminally-caring natures have prevented us from setting appropriate limits, and to make the changes necessary to ensure our very survival? *I am certain that we do.*

If our image has been maligned by male-dominated professions, how have we appeared to other professional women? If the doctors have viewed us as weak, have we also looked weak to our own gender? The feminist movement may have respected the initiative of nursing's founder, but nursing today has not yet been widely supported by women in positions of power.

It seems as if the 'masculine approach' to nursing, the highly technical care, has been recently viewed as much more important than the gentle caregiving, which has consistently gone to less educated and trained caregivers. However, there are thousands of us today preparing, through certification programs and advanced degrees, to use energetic healing methods in our nursing endeavors.

So far, we have had to use our hands and hearts quietly, most often not even charting the special nursing care we give (making it difficult to document the efficacy of our endeavors). Is there not a place for the advanced caring potential that only highly-educated nurses can provide?

Intensive Care nurses command higher salaries and much more respect than our sisters in geriatric facilities, thus causing more nurses to be attracted to this work. Yet, the rapidly-expanding older population in our society requires vastly comprehensive and sensitive caring. Is not nursing truly a complex and multi-faceted profession, complete with technical and humanitarian aspects of *equal* importance?

Nursing alone uniquely offers compassion and concern for all people as its basis. Whereas medical practice can sometimes exist successfully without caring and nurturing, nursing without caring will never promote health. *Caring is a deeply human need, and nursing exists, in part, to fill that need.*

The Media Portrayal: A Fantasy Perspective

To complete the picture of nursing's confusing image, we can now examine the media portrayal of the nurse. Because of the many problems related to nursing's muddled image these days, a dedicated team of researchers devoted a ten-year study to this topic. Beatrice and Philip Kalisch painstakingly reported the many facets of the nursing's media image in their recent book, *The Changing Image of the Nurse.*[19]

These authors believe that politicians and others in power have been terribly misinformed about nursing's role. According to their study, the 19th-century image of the nurse has two opposing characters. One was the image of the unkempt hag (Sairy Gamp in the Dickens novel), and the other the image of the high-class 'saint' (Florence Nightingale). These seem strikingly similar to our actual history, in that nursing went directly from the nuns to the prostitutes and drunks. (*What other profession can boast of such diversity in its ranks?*)

In the silent film era, the nursing role was influenced by a late Victorian morality code. The nurse's image was almost always projected in relation to a man. A positive, upbeat doctor's-handmaiden stereotype typified the movie view of nursing's connection with World War II. During the '30s and prior to World War II, nursing seemed to be portrayed as a noble way for women to earn money. Nurses were shown as competent and trustworthy.

The nurse's work increased even more during World War II, as we were shown to be patriots and valuable contributing members of society. The post-war portrayal, however, found nursing reduced to a dependent position once again. On the screen, nurses seemed to have lost ground in the '60s, becoming the brunt of sexually-suggestive scripts. It became worse in the '70s when nurses were portrayed as malevolent and sadistic, the shadow of a prominent male figure at best.

The Kalisch team clearly demonstrated that a severe setback occurs whenever the nursing role is linked to sexually suggestive material. Male doctors have more intimate knowledge of human anatomy and physiology, yet are much less often portrayed as sex objects. This is merely one example of institutionalized sexual stereotyping of women.

In an article entitled "Hollywood Nurses: A Muddled American Image",[20] Scott W. Shiffer, BSN, contends that nurses are "the front line liaison between the consumer and the health care system . . . the key contributors to health promotion".

Interestingly, according to Mr. Shiffer, the television nurse was not the same as the one shown in the movies. In the '50s, nurses were obviously subordinate to doctors in such popular shows as Ben Casey and Dr. Kildare. The '60s showed nurses increasing their strength on television, but in the '70s nursing again seemed to take a giant leap backwards.

Today, nurses have been uniting to extinguish these silly, inaccurate portrayals of who we are. It is now up to us to articulate our role, and to stop allowing ourselves to be defined by the fantasies of corporate men trying to sell sex, or diminish our worth.

Summary

It has been difficult for nursing to forge ahead in leadership roles and make its valuable contributions to society in the face of such poor media portrayal. Not only do nurses lose something wonderful, but so do American health care consumers.

Each and every nurse can make a difference. Speak up. Write letters. It is up to us to do our part to help clarify the image of nursing in the public eye. Then, and only then, will we regain our collective voice, and perform our special role in health care. *Then* we will recapture the lost art of nursing.

PART II

WHAT IS THE PROBLEM?

———

'SICK CARE' VS HEALTH CARE

Introduction

The following three chapters are personal stories. Each of these describes some painful, yet valuable, experiences with the distinct purpose of further awakening the conspiracy.

Chapter Three is the story of a courageous health care consumer. Chapter Four tells of a young doctor's disillusionment with medical training, and Chapter Five is a collage of my early experiences in the world of nursing.

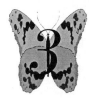

THROUGH THE MILL
A Hero's (and Heroine's) Journey

NOTE: This chapter was written by Loi Eberle, M.A. It is intended to document the journey of a man determined to challenge cancer according to his personal beliefs and desires. It is also the story of those closest to him, and what they learned from this shared journey.

Loi Eberle, M.A. designed and produced instructional media in a variety of university and corporate settings, including the Schools of Allied Health Sciences at the University of Minnesota, before forming a non-profit corporation with her husband Rob Eberle. Through their corporation, they produced and distributed video documentaries, motivational workshops, and written materials, to inspire healing.

It took a while for me to grasp the full impact of the words spoken to me by the nurse who was conducting my health evaluation. "You never have to develop cancer" she told me. It was so liberating to entertain that thought, especially with my family history of cancer.

This nurse at Kaiser Permanente in Oakland, California, was offering me the first opportunity to discuss my fears, and she empowered me to believe in my ability to avoid serious health problems. I had already begun to heal my ulcers and colitis through Yoga and vegetarianism, but up to that point I had questioned whether a person had any control over something as ominous as cancer or heart disease. Since then, I have reflected many times on her words, and the inspiration they offered.

The time was the late '70s, and the idea that nutrition or attitude would affect one's health was considered ludicrous. I worked at a prestigious university science institute, and was watching colleagues die of cancer there. It seemed that science was still grasping for answers, but was not totally open to new input. It was this searching that led me to attend workshops about alternative healing.

One such workshop I attended was offered by a charismatic man named Rob, who spoke about how you can affect your reality through your thoughts, even when your reality includes cancer. He described the long progression of events that led finally to his cancer surgeries - the long-term exposure to radiation from the radar screens in the military, the high stress he experienced participating in a war he didn't believe in, and lifestyle excesses that he indulged in as coping mechanisms. He told of over twenty oral surgeries, misdiagnoses and treatments, and a cross-country quest that eventually led him to a West Coast university medical center.

Rob shared with us what he had learned from participating in support groups with others who had cancer; the striking similarities

58

in their experiences; and the correlations he saw between their attitudes, lifestyles, and outcomes. He talked about how he was learning to de-condition his disease-promoting beliefs. He also spoke
strongly of his frustration at having his insights and therapeutic
choices discounted by group leaders and medical professionals.

A powerful and persuasive speaker, he conveyed his strong
desire to help people heal, and had a great impact on his audience.
After that workshop, I wanted to hear more, and soon found myself
wanting to help him tell his story, and the stories of many others who
were finding their means to health outside the current standard of
medical practice.

Rob had recently undergone two surgeries to remove his max-
illa and the palate in his mouth, in order to rid him of cancer. At that
point, his doctors and pathologists determined there were 'no mar-
gins', that is, the cancer was found right up to the incision. Conse-
quently, it was recommended that he undergo further surgery to
remove his eye and part of his face, and/or receive radiation therapy.

When he discussed the recommendation for radiation with the
specialist who fit him with his oral prosthetic, the man described
how often he saw radiation destroy the salivary glands, causing
fungus disease, and eventually the loss of teeth, making it impossible
to wear a prosthetic appliance. Without the appliance, Rob spoke in
a way similar to a person with cleft palate, and experienced great
difficulty in eating and drinking. Although his doctors vehemently
insisted that he undergo these procedures, and offered dire warnings
about his prognosis without them, no one guaranteed success, or
produced anyone who was successfully recovering with such an
approach.

Rob had already undergone twenty previous dental reconstructive surgeries in the military, and they had left psychological scars. After initially discovering degeneration in his left maxillary sinus during root canal work, his dentist performed reconstructive surgery. To recuperate, he was ordered by his dentist to have a large dose of complete bed rest.

Instead of being able to rest, however, he was immediately ordered back to his instructors' position by a higher authority, thus damaging his surgery and necessitating further reconstruction. He felt that by following the orders from his superior officer, he compromised his recovery and underwent a great deal of pain and stress.

At the end of his time in the service, he was encouraged to sign up for another tour of duty because it was felt the reconstruction work was defective and needed to be completely redone. That, to him, added insult to injury, since he was experiencing extreme anxiety about teaching pilots bombing strategies that could kill innocent people. He chose not to sign on for further military involvement, choosing instead to work in his family's real estate business, hoping to never have to 'take orders' again.

The entire surgical experience had been traumatic for him, and he was vehemently opposed to further cancer surgery and its resulting disfiguration, believing that the success rate was questionable. Feeling he could not live with the options offered, he decided to find another way. His decision started him on a journey that led him to explore a whole new world of healing options. He wanted to share this knowledge as he learned about it.

Rob and I decided to work together to develop workshops and educational videotapes. He had amassed a large number of books about healing and alternative cancer therapies. He wanted to learn more about these therapies and the people who were having success with them. He also wanted to further change his 'limiting belief systems', ideas that he felt stood in the way of his healing process.

We learned more and more about immunotherapy, reading and talking to everyone we could find who had experience with it. He introduced me to his friend Frank who had been sick with class 4 lymphoma. An incorrect medicine raised his temperature up to 105 degrees. Afterwards, he felt better than at any time since his diagnosis. He felt it burned the cancer cells out somehow. He refused further treatments, and a year later was doing fine. *(P.S. - still is, ten years later)*.

Meanwhile, he and Rob watched with great dismay as the rest of the people in his support group sickened and died from the standard cancer therapies they were using. Could temperature manipulation be as helpful to others as it had been to Frank? Was temperature a part of immunotherapy?

Rob felt compelled to share what he was learning. He felt people were suffering and dying unnecessarily. We began to network with holistically-orientated doctors, nurses, and health professionals to develop and teach workshops about cancer recovery.

Some good can come out of any situation. At this juncture, a very negative contact with a medical doctor produced an ally - a wonderful nurse named Marie, who soon became our partner and workshop co-leader. She had worked with Dr. Carl Simonton,[21] alternative cancer specialist, in his early years of using visualization and imagery to overcome cancer. Now she was a nurse specializing in preventive medicine, health education, and alternative healing. How wonderful! I began to think differently about the nursing profession.

The three of us spent many hours developing the workshop content, which we then shared with other nurses and health professionals, also eliciting their feedback and response. Our workshops, which were offered on a donation basis, were well attended.

The workshops contained many emotionally-charged moments. People couldn't understand why doctors would not be receptive to these therapies when a variety of patients were obviously having positive results with them. Their constant questioning caused us to discuss the political ramifications, including information about why the known dangers of many products and chemicals were being withheld from the American public.

It was disturbing to be the ones to shatter people's illusions of security, both with their therapies and with their government. We felt, however, that it was an issue of life and death. During this period, I went to see my dentist. As the hygienist cleaned my teeth, she told me about a man she cared for who had discovered a tumor similar to Rob's. After the diagnosis was confirmed, her client pursued alternative therapies, and was having tremendous success without having to undergo surgery. I told Rob and we met with him.

We realized instantly that we wanted to videotape this man's story to show in our workshops. We felt it was vital for people to hear these stories directly from the source. We did not want to promote any particular therapies, only to show that healing was possible. Thus, we were led to find ways to obtain video equipment to produce a series about cancer alternatives and 'ideal role models' - people who are taking charge of their own healing.

At the same time, we met a woman who was attending Joseph Campbell's[22] classes. She shared with us the importance of myths and legends, and how they have shaped our collective psyche throughout time. We learned about the myth of the hero and his journey to enlightenment, his return, and his sharing it with others. Rob felt that the road to healing was itself a hero's journey. He wanted to document people in various stages of the journey, to excite them about sharing their success with others, not only to inform them, but to inspire the healing process in each 'hero' whose story was in the making.

Rob, Marie and I leased some basic video equipment and my background in instructional media greatly facilitated this process. Interestingly, we found a similarity in the stories of all the interviewees - every time any of them had experienced some sort of healing, their experience was invalidated and discounted by their doctors. There was absolutely no support given for doing anything other than following doctors orders, even when those orders did not produce positive results.

Many workshop attendees were nurses. They had witnessed the grim reality of allopathic medical cancer cures, and were eager to learn if there were alternatives that offered enhanced quality of life. The more we interacted with nurses, the more we realized how stressful were their working conditions. We also found it empowering to receive validation from these nurturing health practitioners. We learned so much from them. Most notable was a dynamic group of nurses in the San Francisco Bay Area, known as Nurses in Transition. Marie was very involved with this group, and invited Rob and I to join them during a retreat to facilitate their incorporation process.

While there, we met Karilee, whose need to conspire had let to the birth of Nurses in Transition. She seemed to be a dynamic and insightful woman who brought her new baby and shared stories about her home birth. She invited us to meet Richard, her husband, who was the co-founder of perhaps the first holistic clinic in the country. We were deeply excited to meet this couple, even though at the time we had no idea as to how many times they would offer us strength, validation, and sound advice.

It was fortunate that we had this kind of support system. It gave us the encouragement we needed to deal with another system, the Veteran's Administration, or VA, that seemed either unable or unwilling to respond to the individual. Rob had been living on disability benefits for his cancer, which had been determined to be a 100% service-connected disability. He was very grateful to receive these benefits, which alleviated the stress of having to support himself. It also enabled him to offer his services for donations only. Eventually, I decided to leave my position as a curriculum evaluator and training program developer to pursue our work together full-time. It was necessary that we adjust to living at his poverty level.

One day Rob was extremely upset by a letter he received from the VA informing him that his 100% benefits would be cut to a mere fraction. They reasoned that if he didn't follow a standard cancer therapy, then he must not have cancer, and was no longer entitled to full benefits. We appealed to the medical authorities, but there was no support for Rob in his pursuits of low-cost, non-invasive therapies, even though success was unproven with the treatment the VA would recognize.

Rob felt their decision violated his freedom of choice to pursue whatever therapy he wanted, even if that meant no therapy. To him, the benefits did not pay for the therapy, but were instead to compensate him for his service-connected disability. Only one doctor, Richard (who had been involved in award winning undergraduate cancer research at University of Pennsylvania Medical School) was willing to support us by writing letters to validate Rob's program of immunotherapy.

During the stress surrounding this predicament, Rob's tooth became badly decayed after losing a filling. He kept requesting an appointment with the VA, but the scheduling kept being postponed. Finally he lost his temper with them on the phone. At that point the clerk admitted that his file was unobtainable because it was trapped, closed by another file cabinet moved in front of it because the office was being painted! By the time Rob got treated, his tooth had to be pulled.

Rob was infuriated by his treatment. He spoke to a VA counselor who among other things discovered that Rob's computer record showed him as having lung cancer, rather than oral cancer. The counselor told him privately that he should fight for his case, to help not only himself, but for the many other veterans he's seen who were too old and sick to fight for their rights. Rob channeled his frustration into writing an excellent appeal to the VA. He visited his congressman, who was extremely upset about how Rob was being treated. It was perhaps this congressman's letter that finally got the VA's attention. Soon Rob was ordered to undergo a medical examination.

It was memorable. The doctor at one point wanted to palpate his surgical site. Rob maintained that one could see his nerve tissue through a paper-thin membrane in the orbit of his eye. Rob refused to let him insert instruments into that area, believing that the slightest false move could cause serious damage. The doctor tried to encourage him, offering to put procaine on his instrument swabs. In his report, the doctor called Rob uncooperative. Eventually, his benefit

65

continuation request was denied. It was on the basis of this physician's visual examination that the VA determined that Rob did not have cancer. Rob continued to maintain that in the past it was only the microscopic pathology report that verified his cancer, that it could not be confirmed by visual examination.

The VA maintained that Rob's immunotherapy was not valid, and that since he was not undergoing therapy, he did not have cancer. Throughout all this, we were working on our own healing, and working on ourselves - to de-program ourselves from the belief systems that caused stress, anger and hostility, and thus, dis-ease. During this time, we encountered a variety of reactions from people, sometimes intense and hostile. We experienced the angry resistance shown by people to the idea that we can trust our own healing ability.

People struggled to maintain their position of subservience to doctors, not daring to trust in the ability of the body to heal. The way we saw it, standard therapies by their very nature compromised the body's functioning. We were intently focused on how to strengthen the body to allow for healing.

The medical model taught people to listen to authorities outside themselves; not to their own internal wisdom. In our belief, by accepting this domination, people see themselves as powerless victims. Taking control of their healing seemed to imply some responsibility for the illness, which people felt was a threatening and self-flagellating concept (to us, it was empowering).

We tried to acquaint them with the notion that 'responsibility' is the 'ability to respond'. One could choose to see responsibility as the recognition of the way in which one's own actions influence one's state of health or disease. This understanding was not to be used to 'blame the victim', but rather to give insight into what a

66

person might need to change in order to promote one's own recovery.

We began to speak to a wide variety of health-related groups in the San Francisco Bay Area. We formed a non-profit organization whose mission was to network the healing endeavors of other groups by offering organizational skills and communication support. Our goal was to further our understanding of 'Psycho-Physical Ecology', a word I coined to describe the study of the interaction between the psyche, the body, and the environment. Many groups were interested in our insights, and Rob's uncanny ability to perceive the 'blind spots' in a given situation.

Once again, Rob lost his appeal to the VA to renew his benefits. We then appealed that decision, with letters, pictures of the extent of his disability, and pathology reports. It was a distinct disadvantage, in these appeals, that Rob was doing amazingly better with his cancer than almost anyone else with the same kind of tumor. Dr. Shames wondered if the pressure to win the appeal might subconsciously force Rob not to do so well with his immunotherapy program. I wondered too, about the repercussions from constantly maintaining that he had cancer, but receiving no benefits because he remained symptom-free.

We continued, in the meantime, to expand our workshop content, producing slide shows and videotapes about healing. As people began to learn of our work, we were invited to present to various groups all over California. The end result was a two hour documentary which we made at my Alma Mater in the Midwest, where we obtained permission to use their production studios during the night (when no one else was there).

We lived in our van, scraping frost off the ceiling over our heads when we awoke in the morning. Around that time, we got married and I became pregnant. With scant resources, we journeyed south, interviewing health practitioners, meeting recovering people, and frequently showing our tape to people very much in need of hope.

In the meantime, we were encountering another aspect of the medical system. I couldn't find a doctor who would give me prenatal care unless I committed to having him be the attending physician in a hospital birth. On the advice of my nurse-friend in San Francisco, I began to compile my own prenatal records. I finally located a doctor who agreed to see me, but when we notified him that we were planning a home birth, he refused treatment. We finally decided to relocate back to southern California, where a midwife who cared for our friends there agreed to do the delivery.

The birth was a wonderful experience, gently guided by midwives and friends. One of the friends attending had been a speaker at a meeting where Rob and I had also presented the year before. At that time, she and her husband had shared the sad story of their daughter.

The child, at a very early age, had developed a rare and deadly form of cancer after being exposed to milk and meat from cows who had been mistakenly fed pesticide-riddled grain, an incident which received national attention at the time. Her chemotherapy treatments were so painful that she would try to scratch at her mother to avoid them. Finally, the parents surrendered to the child's demands, and stopped bringing her for treatments.

Their doctor obtained a court order forcing them to submit their child to chemotherapy or lose custody of her. They felt that chemotherapy was intolerable to the child, given that the prescribed treat-

68

ment was admitted by the AMA to be an experimental drug. They chose to take her to Mexico instead, to receive an alternative, more easily tolerated therapy.

The child survived longer than expected on the new therapy, even improving at first. Although physically comfortable, she was eventually consumed with homesickness, and seemed to give up. She died slowly. In the weeks before my own child was born, I found it unspeakably tragic to think of losing one.

We liked to describe Will's birth as arriving in a circle of angels; nurturing, empowering women - midwives, friends, and a nurse. It was an awe-inspiring event, and I was in bliss around the arrival of our son.

Though we would have preferred to stay home with our new baby, many people were reaching out to us by then for help with their cancer. We continued our video production work. Rob continued to fund-raise and brainstorm new programs. I worked vigorously alongside him, with Will lying in a basket next to me as I edited endless miles of tape.

The financial pressures mounted as we now lived in an affluent area. My menses had not resumed, which I attributed to heavy nursing. However, I soon discovered I was pregnant again. All these factors weighed heavily upon us, and we both felt ready for some of our own healing. We yearned to be in the woods, away from the constant pressure of raising money for expensive video productions.

It was around this time that we received word that our VA appeal had been offered a hearing in Washington, D.C. Rob's testimony at that hearing was very impressive. I testified as well, describing some of the basis in literature for immunotherapy. I felt Rob had made a strong argument, as did many others who later read the transcript from the hearing. It would be a while before we would hear the verdict.

We travelled in search of a nest for our family, feeling the pressure of being on the road and pregnant. Just in time, we located a midwife in the Northwest, who assisted us with the wonderful birth of our second son, Adam. Through her, we met many of the midwives in this region, all of whom were intelligent, knowledgeable, and compassionate healers. These women were deeply concerned about the extreme lack of understanding of the nature and safety of midwifery.

Those early days in the country, amid such beautiful surroundings, were magical. Life was peaceful in the rustic environment, and we relished the contrast from our hectic life of recent months. Adam was a quiet baby; his peaceful countenance affected everyone deeply when they were around him. Several weeks later, I was asked to assist the midwife at a birth. It was profoundly moving to help this beautiful Native American woman birth her fifth son.

Her baby was especially robust, crying vigorously at birth and thereafter, grasping to be suckled. The contrast to my own quiet, sleeping baby was striking. I had an unsettling feeling of sadness, and asked the midwife to check Adam. I had noticed that he seemed to breathe rapidly from time to time.

Based on the midwife's advice, we decided to take the baby to our back-up doctor in a neighboring town. The doctor examined the baby and turned to me: "Your baby is going to die. It could be tomorrow, it could be in three weeks, but he won't live long."

70

He explained to us how Adam's plumbing was wrong. The valve to reverse his blood flow at birth had never closed, and he would require repeated surgeries. He informed us that despite medical intervention, Adam would never live a normal life, or a long life.

He asked us to consider where we wanted to spend the rest of our time with him. He informed us that once we took him to the hospital, we would essentially lose control of his experience and we should consider where we would have the best support systems once we did this. We asked if we had time to take him home first; there were things we needed to do.

After calling and sobbing to Karilee and Rich in California, and much discussion with dear friends, we decided to go a large medical center. We went home to pack, planning to leave first thing in the morning. I had a very difficult time trying to sleep that night. Finally, after dawn, Adam woke to nurse. I offered him my breast and held him close. Snuggling, we drifted off to sleep.

Adam's sharp inhalation woke me suddenly. I shook Rob to tell him Adam was having trouble breathing. He took him in his arms and looked at him. To our horror, we realized that the breath we had heard had been his last. After unsuccessful attempts to revive him, I simply held him, staring at his lifeless form with unspeakable grief. Finally, Rob left to notify the family.

They soon arrived to comfort us, and we decided that we would bury him on the land where we lived. Looking for a plot, Rob and I roamed the land where I had walked so recently, singing to the baby. Every so often we would hold each other and sob.

I sat by my baby and grieved, while Rob dug his grave. I watched how his facial color changed as his life force left him. My mind went on a million different tangents. My parents tried to comfort me as I listened to the sounds of Rob building a coffin out of pine. Friends began to arrive in preparation for the burial.

We all stood silently, stunned by the recent events. Photos of that time show the wide-eyed expressions of the young children. We spoke of Adam's beautiful energy, and wished him well on his journey. We sang a farewell song, said goodbyes, and lowered him into the ground.

The months that followed were agony. At first, I lay on the ground every day next to Adam's grave, feeling like crawling in after him. Finally, one day Rob came out and took me by the shoulders and asked "Which direction are you going in? Toward the living or the dead? What about Will and me?"

It finally sunk in. I saw where I was headed. I began to force myself to make an effort to focus on life. I grieved deeply, but also cooked meals for others, and attended births, celebrating new life.

Although probably I was not easy to be around, I allowed myself the luxury of grief, openly crying when I needed to. Rob, on the other hand, was still susceptible to the male conditioning of our culture. Rather than allowing himself to express the emotion, he intellectualized it, comforting himself with lots of fishing excursions and occasional food binges.

A few months later the real pain set in. A sore appeared at the old surgery site. There had been other signs - mainly a sense of impending doom. When he first told me about the sores, I felt it was a nightmare coming true. Though I tried to be optimistic, terror lurked in the back of my mind.

We began the fasting and dietary changes, making essene bread, rejuvelac, and growing wheat grass at our friend's house. I walked a few miles through the snow to cut and juice the wheat grass (a strenuous and time consuming operation), then I'd hike back to give it to him. Rob insisted on keeping a positive attitude, and became hostile when I tried to express my fears. His pain began to increase.

He could no longer wear his prosthetic device; it's tight fit over his new lesions was too painful. He ate and spoke without it, despite the large hole in his palate and the upper part of his throat. I knew we would have to leave the physically-demanding life we had established, and seek a more comfortable home in town.

We moved in with Rob's sister, and became active in local anti-pesticide spraying endeavors. Rob would speak and submit to the city council summaries of research reports I had compiled from extensive research. I found this work empowering as I endeavored to heal myself of Adam's loss.

Rob decided it was time to approach the VA about those benefits denied because he must not have cancer anymore. He went to a local dentist to have a cast made of the lesions in his mouth. He began to document it in photographs. His intention was to show how his mouth would look as it healed.

We accepted an offer to appear on a television show in Berkeley, California. This gave us a minor opportunity to discuss our experiences. We explored avenues for getting my books and videos produced. We met a film producer who invited me to narrate a television production he was doing about a medical doctor from Chicago who had originated a unique detoxification program.

The more we learned about the body, and chemical contamination, the more we believed in the importance of detoxification. We returned to our rural atmosphere, contacted the physician who specialized in detoxification, and invited him to work with us. We engaged ourselves in building and using colonic machines, fasting, and eating macrobiotically. Rob was showing progressive deterioration, and it was becoming increasingly critical to find a program that would help him. Friends were very supportive, and also were eager to learn to promote their own well-being.

Finally, Rob felt it was time to go to the VA to verify his condition, and to have some support with pain relief. I dreaded going back to a VA hospital. Each time the experience had been extremely depressing. It was a great surprise to be met by a nurse practitioner, Anna, who I later called the 'VA Shaman'. She was the first health professional inside an institution who was at all receptive to Rob's desire to pursue immunotherapy.

Recently, *Newsweek* quoted the National Cancer Institute's chief of surgery, Dr. Steven Rosenberg, as saying "In the coming century, immunotherapy could transform the practice of medicine."[23] However, back then, the VA felt Rob's desire to pursue immunotherapy instead of radiation or chemotherapy was grounds for rescinding his benefits. That same *Newsweek* article described how cancer researchers are "disheartened by the archaic rituals of radiation and chemotherapy". Yet even though there was little evidence that these therapies were effective, the medical professionals continued to pressure Rob to submit to what he described as 'torture'.

Anna didn't pressure; she listened. She heard that Rob wanted his condition verified. He wasn't looking for treatment, he wanted to pursue the therapies he already was using, but felt that at least now they could visually inspect him and see the lesions. He was hopeful that they would now reinstate his benefits, significantly reducing our stress level.

Obviously alternative therapies were not paid for by the VA, nor were they offered in their clinics. We had to buy the vitamins, special foods, build the sauna and colonic machine, etc. with our own money, which was incredibly scarce. In looking back, I wonder how we managed to survive at all. Rob certainly couldn't work, and required my full-time attention as well. We had become accustomed to living in poverty, and felt fortunate to be living in a town where most other people lived simply also.

Anna assessed his vital signs, discussed his condition, and most importantly, listened to what he wanted - why he was there. I am still amazed at what a difference a good nurse can make!

She knew the doctors there, and because she was a nurse practitioner, she could select the doctor to whom she would make her referral. She selected a kindly, grandfatherly man who we learned later was close to retirement. She explained to the doctor Rob's wishes, and also expressed his desire to have assistance with pain control. By then, the pain was so severe that it was becoming difficult for him to keep up the fight.

We left that day with a tremendous feeling of relief. Anna had made a deep impression on us. We knew we had an ally, someone who was finally supportive of Rob's efforts to pursue a personal program of immunotherapy.

Rob was finding some pain reduction through the detoxification procedures we were using. Aside from the pain, he was having a relatively good quality of life. We fasted at times, ate macrobiotically, took saunas and colonics. Even though the tumor growth was slow, Rob's experience was becoming more challenging. We didn't have a lot of guidance about what to do, but could see what was being tried in conventional medicine, and the limited effectiveness it had. Occasionally Anna would call. Her calls were a great comfort, sometimes the only outlet I had for my emotions. She was truly a rock for me.

Eventually we were informed that Rob's 100% benefits were reinstated. It was a great relief, but we felt they should have been granted retroactively, since it was clear we were entitled to them all along. We had to further pursue the fight for retroactive benefits.

Despite our healing efforts, and perhaps exacerbated by our stressful circumstances, the uvula in the roof of Rob's palate was being eaten away. It dangled precariously, and Rob was afraid it would fall down his throat and possibly choke him. We went to the VA to talk to Anna, who brought in a young doctor to work with us - a doctor who was a leader in a local environmental group. He advised us how to handle the situation, and about possible complications, such as bleeding too much from the numerous capillaries.

I was concerned about whether I could leave him alone. One night Rob was in the bathroom for a very long time, and came out presenting me with a square inch piece of flesh on a plate. I felt weak as he described how he had removed it while it was falling out.

After he assured me that he was okay, I still felt shaky. I called Anna, and was extremely grateful to be able to talk to her at that point. That episode prompted us to get more help. We travelled to Boston to receive a family consultation with world-renowned Michio Kushi,[24] a leader in the Macrobiotic movement.

After we followed Kushi's recommendations for several months, during a brief improvement in Rob's condition, I became pregnant.

We were ecstatic, and hopeful. Nine months later, Emily was born after I labored in the bath. The first months of her life passed quickly.

We received notification from the VA that we had been granted a reconsideration before the VA Board of Appeals, after communications with the offices of several senators. (I had spent months bringing attention to Rob's case, because I felt strongly that it was an issue of Freedom of Choice. Friends supported our cause and wrote letters as well.)

The VA had restored Rob's 100% disability benefits as a result of doctor's interviews that had been set up by Anna at the VA. Suddenly, the argument that they hadn't excised all of the tumor the first time, became more persuasive. It was consistent with the current medical concept that increased stress, such as the loss of a child, would greatly intensify a condition that otherwise would be controlled by one's immune system. At any rate, they determined that indeed there had been an error in the factual findings based upon the evidence of the record. They would re-hear our case.

For me, it was good news and bad news. Once again, we would have to leave the beautiful nest I had created, and go on the road. It had been such a magical, yet brief, respite in our little house on the edge of the wooded mountain, where we had birthed our baby girl. Freeways and Washington D.C. bureaucrats did not sound like fun. All the while, Rob's health had continued to deteriorate.

We had some poignant time visiting family, always with lots of laughter. One hour prior to our hearing, we met with the Disabled American Veterans, who were representing our case. After the hearing, we spent Thanksgiving with Rob's parents.

Soon afterward, our forwarded mail informed us of another 'Catch 22' - that the VA computer had been programed years ago to cut off payments as of a certain date. We were told that they couldn't do anything about it unless we produced his file. Yet, in Washington they informed us that if we pulled his file from there, it would be a very long time before the Appeals Board could reach a decision.

Unfortunately, we were so desperately in need of money, we had to request that the file be sent back so we could receive our monthly check, even though it would compromise the potential of $40,000 in retroactive benefits to which we were also entitled. That money certainly could have helped defray the costs of the alternative therapies that Rob so desperately wanted right then. It seemed ludicrous that the VA and insurance would pay for toxic chemicals, but not food, vitamins, and herbs.

At this point, Rob at 5'11", weighed less than 100 pounds. Rob's brother insisted we get more qualified help at an alternative retreat center. Though Rob had originally been given a year and a half to live, it was almost five years later. We were still taking walks together. Anna had shared with me on the phone one day that the specialist told her he had never seen anyone with this tumor, regardless of therapy, live as long as Rob. He also told Anna that whatever we were doing should be supported to the utmost. He felt certain that we were breaking new ground.

I can't tell you how empowering it was to receive these tiny bits of support from inside the system. There were times when, for me, those tiny endorsements gave me the courage to face the next round. I knew it wasn't just for Rob that we continued on this journey.

Rob had a hard time staying on the macrobiotic diet. I blamed

78

the pain killers he was on. Yet, without them, the pain was too intense for him to want to live. They took him out of touch with his intention to use nutritional therapy, and made him susceptible to 'binge foods'. It was terribly frustrating to spend hours making a macrobiotic meal, then learn he had gone out later for pie. It was the big secret he shared with the kids. Though I was upset, I also knew those were probably very bonding times for them. "Who knows how many more there would be," I would rationalize.

In the comfort of a remote retreat center, with healthy meals being prepared and positive role models all around, we felt nurtured. As Rob's condition worsened, he was moved to a nearby facility, which made it more difficult to secure the meals easily. Rob became too weak to walk, due to a painful bowel obstruction and his refusal to eat until his condition was resolved. I realized with terror that I did not have the physical strength to care for all his needs, nurse my baby, and care for my son and myself.

I called Anna. Always there for me, she spent quite a while discussing Rob's current situation. She spoke of the usual procedures performed in a hospital setting for this kind of condition. She even suggested he take his narcotic pain-killers again, as he had stopped them suddenly, two weeks prior, feeling they were not good for him. She described how his system had become dependent upon them to stimulate peristalsis. This explained to us the mass he felt, and lack of bowel activity.

I felt pressured and knew I had to do something. Some people tried to insist that I take him to the hospital. Others reminded me that Rob didn't want to die in a hospital, so why take him there? It was the first time anyone matter-of-factly spoke to me about his death. I had been so imbued with positivism, I figured he would pull out of

79

it, just as he had many times before.

I called the hospital emergency room and asked to speak to the head nurse on duty. I explained Rob's condition, and asked what they would do for him. I asked her, on a very personal level, to please tell me what would normally happen. She told me that in his current state, they certainly wouldn't attempt any invasive procedures, that they could provide bed rest, observation, and basic care. She said that if he refused treatment, they could do nothing unless he were declared legally incompetent.

When I spoke with Rob, he took me by the shoulders, looked intensely into my eyes, and told me he trusted me not to take him there, no matter what. It was a great act of trust (he could not stop me if he wanted to) since by this time he was so emaciated that I could have thrown him over my shoulder and carried him myself!

I asked his brothers to drive out to help. They arrived the next day. Meanwhile I was conflicted with emotion and suggestions. Friends gave Rob acupressure and massage treatments. We gave him ginger baths, with foam pads protecting his protruding bones. I sat next to him in the candle light.

Rob decided he wanted to take a few days to get stronger, then go back home. He also decided to try eating again. That possibility seemed remote, since at that point he could no longer even swallow rice cream baby cereal because of the extent of the decomposition of the throat tissue. However, several days later he announced that he was ready to go home that day. He wrote me a grocery list for junk foods, and told me to get them at the corner store. I asked if he really wanted me to do that. He angrily told me to get them.

I walked to the store, and called Anna from the phone booth in

80

the deeply piled snow. She advised me to get him what he wanted; that he must have his reasons. She spent quite a while talking to me about how to be strong and supportive through all of this. I was upset because Rob seemed to be turning on me, and Anna wisely reminded me that Rob really loved me; that it was his sickness that was causing him to distance himself.

Anna's words gave me courage. I brought the groceries back to the apartment, Rob attempted to eat some of the food, but could not swallow it. I began packing our belongings. Suddenly the shortness of time overwhelmed me. I kneeled next to Rob, and cherished our silent time together. Tears quietly rolled down my cheeks. I meditated and chanted. There seemed to be no need to share words.

Emily crawled into the room and put her head on Rob's shoulder while he lay there on the floor. It broke my heart. Will came in and told him he loved him, and Rob patted him as well. I noticed that one of his eyes was staring off in a slightly different direction than the other. This was new. His friend showed 'emergency pressure points' to stimulate energy. It was time to go.

Six of us picked him up along with the pad he was lying on, and walked down the large stairway. We loaded Rob, our children and myself into his brother's van. My dear friend Marion had been gently caring for Will and Emily, and told Will that Rob would always be with him. I am so grateful to her for her kindness and sensitivity.

It was late at night, and there was an ice-storm going on, glazing the mountain roads. It seemed absurd to be leaving in these conditions. We had been on the road less then twenty minutes when our van slid toward two cars that were spinning out of control on either side of us. I was sure we were all doomed. Unbelievably we

81

glided between them, straightened out, and kept on driving. I started to speak of the miracle when I looked down at Rob, and a smile crossed his face, lighting up his entire countenance. I hugged him and once again, told him how much I loved him. Then I heard a rattle in his throat, and his chest heaved. He never drew another breath.

I knew he was no longer with us. I could find no pulse, or heartbeat. Soon he became stiff. I told his brother that I could find no vital signs, hoping not to let on to my son what that meant. We stopped at the next rest area to inform Rob's parents and call the family mortician. We were instructed to bring Rob to the hospital when we arrived. His brother, who was driving our car, and I stood in front of the phone and cried together.

After all that had transpired, it was such a quiet, unceremonious passing, devoid of words and goodbyes. Yet, Rob had always scoffed at the 'dying' literature, pronouncing that if you knew how to live well, you could die well.

When I got into the van, Will told me that he was afraid that Rob would die. I gently answered, sorrowfully, that Rob did just die. I'll never forget his shrill howl, when he heard the news. We held each other and cried. Will kept questioning the finality of it, hoping that he was only asleep.

Eventually Will fell asleep, and I sat next to Rob's body, burning sage and chanting until we arrived in Rob's home town. We went to the emergency room, where we were told that we would have to wait until Rob could be examined by a doctor. Hours passed, and we kept asking to be helped. Finally a doctor was able to go to the van. I went out first to say my goodbyes. I took a lock from his hair and put it in my medicine bag. It was unspeakable to me that

I would never stroke his hair again.

We went to Rob's mother's house to be in grief together. Soon I had to make decisions about the body. It was beyond me to have to suddenly refer to my husband as 'the body'. And I hated to have to deal with the system that would require an autopsy, to establish cause of death, for future benefits.

I went to the room Rob and I had shared in the basement. I slept, completely exhausted from the experience. I dreamed of Rob hugging me goodbye. Even though our communication was so open, it hurt that he had never said goodbye. Yet he had constantly affirmed that we would always be together. When I awoke, laying there alone in the dark, I saw that I had a choice. I could let this destroy me, and probably my children too, or I could decide that I would be strong and be the survivor that Rob always advocated. I could see how easy it would be to give up.

I decided at that moment that I would somehow let this be a positive experience. I forced myself to reflect on our years together. People were often amazed at how much fun we had together - how much we seemed to enjoy life.

Sure, there were many painful moments, yet even so, Rob was able to die in dignity. He never submitted to the invasive procedures he despised, or suffered any further disfiguration. No heroic measures were used to eke out a few more miserable hours of life, hooked up to machinery. He was always a free spirit, even in his final situation. I felt he was as much in charge as possible, given his circumstances.

So my tears were not for him, as he was in a much deeper peace; they were due to my attachment to his physical form. Even so,

I allowed myself the luxury of expressing them. I also spent a lot of time crying with Will. Emily was always at my side, and seemed to cry constantly.

Anna was one of the first people I called. We cried together, and she comforted me with her Taoist perspective. Talking to her helped me feel a little less lost and alone. I called other friends across the country. My family arrived, and we made funeral arrangements, had a beautiful ceremony, and celebrated together afterwards.

When notified of his death, the VA immediately requested that I send back the benefits I had received that month. There I was at Rob's mothers' house, with two children, no money, thousands of miles away from my home.

After more discussion with the VA, I realized that receiving the additional money to which I felt entitled was virtually hopeless. I did, however, have some hope for receiving social security benefits, though already twice rejected. Despite my traumatized condition, I knew in my heart that I had to get those benefits to be able to raise my children and survive. Another appeals hearing was granted due to new evidence I was able to uncover.

I drove our kids back to the Northwest for the hearing, and I called Anna. She was again a rock of strength for me. I stayed with her and we talked many hours about what we had shared with Rob. The hardest thing for me to deal with was the sense of failure.

I had many bleak moments at first, feeling that Rob and I had lost all our battles. I eventually learned to reframe the idea of death as a failure, and admit that I knew nothing about death and beyond. Rob and I always felt that our consciousness continued after death, in another form. Regardless of the details, I felt that this life was such an awe-inspring miracle, that if there is anything beyond this, it is probably equally miraculous, even surpassing this realm. But even if there is nothing more, his experience can stand on its own.

I kept reminding myself about how many happy times Rob and I had shared, even in the midst of suffering. We had learned to appreciate and relish the most mundane of moments for the miracle they were. And he *had* lived many years longer then he had been expected to live.

I thought, too, about our experience with baby Adam. I felt comforted by the incredible peace we had shared together. His life had never been traumatized by experimental procedures. Ironically, during the same time that we were dealing with baby Adam's passing, there was a lot of press about Baby Doe receiving an ape's heart for the same condition.

Baby Doe died, after repeated surgeries, on the cold metal operating table. Baby Adam died in my arms, after peacefully nursing to his fill. There is something very empowering about participating in birthing and dying as part of the human family, rather then as a cog in a giant machine.

I felt grateful that I could be with Rob and Adam, without having to be tormented by procedures that would only cause them misery, procedures with slim chances of effectiveness. Later research had shown me that usually they wait for a year before attempting surgery on a baby in Adam's condition - because if they can't live that long, they aren't strong enough to undergo the surgery.

And what if Rob had allowed himself to undergo the entire medical route? He would have had to deal with much more disfigurement, disempowerment, and extreme discomfort. We never did

85

hear of anyone with Rob's type of tumor who had survived those procedures for any length of time.

And what if he had followed the alternative healing modalities more faithfully? I had met people who had long outlived their prognosis using these therapies, though proponents are quick to say that while they had improved the quality of life, they couldn't guarantee increased longevity.

I suppose that what we really want when a loved one is dying is for the person to have an improved quality of life, to be honored for who they are, and to have a respectful environment in which to experience the powerful insights and deepening wisdom that illness provides.

It still hurts to read about the current success in the reversal of chronic conditions through the use of diet, nutrition, exercise, yoga, and meditation. It is very unfortunate that such alternatives were not given any credibility, or even any serious study, until recently.

I think of Rob's passion to share the message about how our body is designed to heal. "Give it what it needs and it will re-stabilize and revitalize."

It has become lucrative to take away people's faith in themselves and in the natural order of life, and instead assign power and authority to technology. Women are afraid to trust their bodies to the birth process. People have lost faith in their ability to tap into energies we know exist - the very energies that could inspire their immune systems to heal them - just because medical science has been unable/unwilling to define them.

Fortunately there are compassionate ones, often (in my experience) the nurses, who have always supported people in finding their own strength and sources of healing. By receiving the gift of who they are, and acknowledging their powerful role in the healing process, they can help their clients and themselves throw off the oppressive authoritarian denial of the true nature of their healing. With their strength and confidence, they can support their clients' journey to health, or help them find meaning in their journey beyond.

Again and again I have had to eschew the notion of death as failure. The more I read about near-death experiences, and the more I reflect on conversations Rob and I shared, the more comfort I feel in Rob's choice to 'drop his body'.

And I often think of that beautiful smile I saw on his face. He looked so peaceful in death. I realized that my sense of loss is my issue. I think his passing was really his graduation. At least, I prefer to think about it that way . . .

And as for the nurses, I give thanks from the bottom of my heart for each gentle touch that helped me to find my own strength and courage during so many trying times. *There are no words to define that healing presence, the loving support, and the feminine form of strength that nurses so quietly possess. You are beacons of light.* It is so often to you, who become truly an extension of our family - the human family - that we entrust our loved ones for help, hope, and healing. I honor you.

Postscript

Since Rob's death, Loi had devoted her time to raising their two children, midwifery advocacy, co-founding and operating a Waldorf-inspired alternative school, teaching yoga, and showing her watercolor and acrylic paintings in regional juried shows.

An Epilogue from Loi

After reading the proofs for this book, I got in touch with the frustration I was so often filled with during Rob's healing journey. I feel so much in agreement with what has been written in this book about healing; so did Rob. So why did he die?

I saw that I had to caution myself (again) about taking a simplistic view of disease, including the variety of ways it affects the psyche. Likewise, I realized that I'm still conditioned to view disease in terms of a win/lose scenario. When we do that, we don't even begin to grasp the full implications of what disease means for our body, mind, spirit & environment. It certainly is a great teacher.

I continue to describe Rob's experience as a healing journey. Though the result was death, immeasurable healing took place. Rob's insights offer a profound wisdom for every person on such a journey, regardless of their particular path.

Our culture is fixated on 'winning', with death as the unavoidable loss. I can't make judgements for Rob about whether the outcome of his experience was positive or negative. It is not that clearly defined, and to be forced by our technologically-orientated medical consciousness to make such 'right/wrong' distinctions about disease, treatment, even life and death, does not take into account the bigger picture. I suspect death is merely another passage in a much longer journey.

What I do know is that Rob's presence in our midst, and the insights he gained as a result of his disease, have had profound implica-

tions for many people. This is not a loss! Should anyone be inspired to be more medically assertive after reading his story, his spirit lives on even that much more . . .

End.

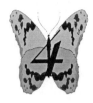

MEDICINE MAN
One Doctor's
Heartfelt Transformation

NOTE: This chapter was written by Richard L. Shames, M.D. It has been added to broaden the concept of conspiracy by demystifying the 'medical mindset' and encouraging more doctors to join nursing's efforts to put the caring back into curing.

Richard L. Shames M.D. is a health educator, author and father. A graduate of Harvard College and University of Pennsylvania, he has served in various capacities ranging from researcher at the National Institutes of Health to clinic doctor at a small county health department. In the 1970's, he founded and directed one of the country's first holistic health centers. He is presently a family physician in private practice in Mill Valley, California. This story describes the turning point in his medical career.

"If this guy would just die already, then maybe I could get some sleep tonight." Imagine me thinking that. Here I was on top of him, using my clasped hands to pump on his heart.

His name was Jay Fitz, a 46-year old red-haired father of three. He had arrived by ambulance, sweating heavily, clutching his chest, and looking very afraid. Five minutes later he was unconscious.

"What have we got now?" I asked between pumps.

"We've got nothing," said Larry. "This damn machine is no good." The monitor had stopped working and the nurses frantically searched for another one. It was a dramatic effort, intense, full of energy, and from my view one big pain.

Last night I had been up working all night long. I'd worked all today without a break. Now I was working again tonight, filling in for another intern who was sick. I was very, very tired.

I was going to be around the whole next day, plus I had a case to present to the chief. If this guy didn't die I might be up half the night, totally consumed with caring for him.

"Get the paddles ready. We'll probably have to shock him." I sounded concerned, but mainly I was angry. I was angry at him for having a heart attack and for having the bad grace to come in right at this moment, when everything else in the hospital was quiet. I had worked myself into exhaustion handling all of my I.V.'s, all of my stomach tubes, all of my major injections and chart work. I had gotten it all done, and here it was, 12:30 a.m. Maybe time to get a little sleep.

Here was Fitz, in danger of dying. And who was going to save him? A young doctor in training, who wanted him to die.

Even then I realized there was something important about this.

92

I had never wanted anybody to die before. It was inconceivable. I had gone into medicine because I wanted people to live, to be healthy. I was always considered a caring person, very sensitive, sympathetic and understanding. Maybe I should have been a nurse.

"Ventricular fibrillation!" shouted Larry from the new EKG.

"Just what I thought. Hand me the paddles." A flick of my thumb sent 400 volts across his chest. For the moment his heart went back into normal sinus rhythm. I was surprised to hear myself thinking: "Come on, Jay, call it quits, already - let me get a few hours sleep tonight."

Something was dreadfully wrong with the medical system in which I was being trained. This man's life was entrusted to some young medical professional who, for want of sleep, was no longer functioning like a human being. I hated to see myself this way - uncivilized and animalistic. The many subterranean discontents that had been brewing in me for years now came shooting to the surface. There was just too much that was absolutely unsavory about the "art of medicine" as presently practiced. I suddenly realized that I was going to do something about it.

This moment where Jay Fitz's life hung in the balance would be the turning point.

Jay eventually died, but he didn't die quickly. I had to stay up most of the night and take care of him in the CCU, only to have him die a few days later, after being transferred to a medical ward. I'd heard that half the people who have heart attacks die whether or not they get to a doctor. Many of them die very quickly so they never get to the hospital. Many others get to the hospital, and then they die. And none of it seems to matter very much, the equipment, the medicines, what the doctors do - they die anyhow.

The same thing happened to my father back East a few months later. He made it to the hospital in a rescue van, which got to him within a couple of minutes. He died anyway. Maybe he died because the intern who was there was just as tired and crazy from lack of sleep as I was. So my father died, Fitz died, and a series of changes had begun for me.

Some were very major changes. I knew that first I had to change myself. I couldn't face what I had become. If successful here, then maybe I could tackle the system.

One surgical nurse I had met was already doing that. Bella would talk about her "consciousness raising group" and their efforts to upgrade health care. Maybe that wasn't as bad an idea as I had first thought. Clearly, the nurses had some bright ideas. They covered the hospital in eight-hour shifts. Even students could get regular sleep. By comparison, my working all day and all night and all the next day was a dumb plan. Maybe a lot of the way medicine was structured was equally dumb.

When I would share these ideas with colleagues, I'd get back crooked disapproving smiles. Most had a lot of respect for the system. They felt that modern American medicine is the greatest anywhere in the world; that it is the pinnacle of scientific achievement. There was a lot of mutual patting on the back about what a great job we were doing, what masters we were over life and death.

To me, it didn't seem that way at all. I sensed that whether the person died, got worse, or got better, it was often between the person and the illness. The doctors were just there doing an elaborate tribal dance. If the person got better they took credit for it. If the person didn't get better they said there was nothing they could do anyway. It was in God's hands.

I became haunted with this image of medicine men dancing around the campfire, shaking a rattle and doing a chant in a strange, mysterious tongue. The dance was now around the bedside, chanting to other doctors in unintelligible medical jargon. The nurses would have to come in after the doctors left to translate and reassure. And huge machines would be wheeled in, completing the scene with an impressive array of technological rattles.

The hypothermia blanket was such a machine. It could bring a person's body temperature down five or six degrees and was fueled by a big silver box that rattled a lot. The cardiac monitors were great rattles with their 'bleep-bleep-bleep'. There were portable x-ray machines that could be wheeled to the bedside. Everyone standing around the bed would do a little bit more of a dance, and the machine would always rattle. Everything from the food carts to the ultrasound machine had Walter Mitty's 'pockata-pockata' rattle. These sounds were easy to get used to and tune out, but as I began to listen freshly, they took on aspects of a strange, futuristic ritual dance.

There were also lots of rattles that we carried around with us. The little syringes for drawing blood would always rattle. So would the symbol of our doctorhood, the ubiquitous stethescope. The more you used it, the more of a doctor you were. If you just listened to the heart you were pretty much of a novice. If you listened also to the lungs and abdomen you were at least a doctor. But if you used it in addition to listen to the carotid artery and hepatic vein, then you were getting pretty good. Here and there you could one-up your colleagues by placing the stethescope over some obscure place on the body and pretend great diagnostic subtlety. The stethescope was a

95

great rattle.

I guess I was becoming a bit obsessed with the image. But in the long hours of making the rounds when my mind would get into some interesting places from lack of sleep, I would fantasize about medicine men and pretend I was one.

I'd have a bone in my nose, a pony tail, a rattle, a set of masks, and a deep, mysterious gaze. A member of the tribe comes to see me for some complaint and sits down on a rock. I peer, gaze, poke, punch, meditate, chant, and suddenly I've got it! I leap up and disappear into the back room of my office, which is a mud hut where there are rows and rows of masks: fearful masks, sad masks, happy masks, and ferocious masks. I quickly find just the right mask, put it on, tiptoe silently out the back, come up from behind the patient, and let out a 'whoop'. The patient turns around, sees the mask, has some appropriate experience, and is instantly much better. Medicine man takes off the mask. The patient, now relaxed and healed, bows and pays me two lizards.

Different cultures, different styles. Perhaps, we in modern fast-changing America haven't yet had time to perfect our rituals. Although we've got our own dance, rattle, and mystery, we may not be sure of what is really effective and what is not.

Take the case of heart conditions. The essence of the therapy that works for heart attacks is simple rest - putting the patient back to bed. You may think that what we're doing for heart attacks is awesomely complex, with all the drugs and machines. The essence of the therapy, however, is that if someone has a heart attack you put him to bed. So what about our fancy Coronary Care Units? A series of articles in the British Medical Journal, *Lancet*, seriously questioned their usefulness. For some patients, they may simply be an expensive part of the ritual.

The truth, in my opinion, is that modern Western medicine is still in a primitive state. We don't have a cure for cancer, heart disease, schizophrenia, diabetes, arthritis, AIDS, or stroke. We can't even cure the common cold. Nevertheless we revel in all sorts of barbarous potions and surgeries.

The tribal medicine man was perhaps less primitive. A subtle psychologist, he knew how to tune into the lives of his tribesmen and elicit suitable emotional responses when needed. He was acquainted with dreams and symbolism. Often healer and healee would sit and face each other, go into a trance, and have a chance to work out what might have been the ultimate cause of the disease. He also knew how to direct the energies of his village in dances and rituals, where the individuals would lose for a time their personal identities and merge with the intense group energy. All this could have a deep and powerful healing effect.

The doctors in the hospital where I was working seldom took anything into account other than the immediate physical process at hand. They neglected the patient's relationship to himself, his family, and his community. No connection was seen between health and spiritual well being. The kind of food the patients ate, the way they exercised, the way they dealt with stressful situations - none of this was even remotely considered by the medicine men of our strange, lopsided, hospital culture.

Sitting and talking with the patients any more than 'absolutely necessary' was a social taboo. Once I was told by Cal, my resident, "Rich, you're spending too much time with your patients." Taken aback, I asked him what he meant. He said, "Listen, you're spending an hour in there taking that history and doing that physical. You've got too much else to do than to waste time like that. You go in there, do that history in ten minutes, do the physical in five, and then get your rear-end out of there."

I protested that it takes longer than that to hear what the people have to say. But Cal was unshakable: "Rich, what they have to say is baloney. You don't want to know what they have to say. You just want to know what's physically wrong with them."

Cal was only one year further along than I. Yet here he was in charge of my medical training, at least the eight weeks of my internal medical rotation.

Was he simply a crass, rude pipsqueek? Was he just a social ignoramus that had learned a lot of science? Yes, and in addition he was echoing what the older attending physicians and house staff would have said. No doctors at our hospital spent time talking with the patients. There was too much else to do than to waste time finding out 'why' someone was sick and 'what' the illness meant to their life. There was hardly even time for words of comfort or sincere encouragement. That was left to the nurses, as if it wasn't really an important job.

It seemed similar to the way the junior resident got the job of sewing the skin back up, after the important surgery was done. I began to wonder if comfort and encouragement might be for some people the most important job. The nurses must have thought so. They always seemed to try to make time for it.

The problem was that even if Cal and the others did have plenty of time, they would not be inclined toward that sort of emotional investment anyway. Therefore it was taboo in my circles.

I sensed that it was somewhat primitive to neglect emotional

98

and spiritual factors in health care. Yet there was great pressure on me to do just that. All the mindless ordering, charting, requisitioning, and case presenting were really quite important to me.

Fundamentally, this was how I would be evaluated. The written word counted for a great deal, while the quality of care, being abstract and difficult to measure, was not given much consideration. And of course getting a good evaluation was of supreme importance, just as it had been since early in high school.

Do well at high school to get into a good college. Be impressive there, because the competition for med schools is fierce. The better you do at med school, the more prestigious an internship you will get. A favorable evaluation here would allow you another good hospital for residency. With a good residency you could then get good post-doctoral fellowship training. Then you might go and become an assistant professor somewhere . . . and up and up and up. The patients were sometimes an annoying distraction along the climb to success. Being a thoughtful, caring doctor was not encouraged. Instead, you wrote good reports, presented impressive cases, and knew all the journal articles. Eventually your advancement and prestige would be based on how many journal articles you could get published.

The day after Fitz died, I had made up my mind. One way to change myself into less of a barbarian would be to cease this endless climbing. If I were no longer concerned about being evaluated for the next step, then I'd be free - free to become a new kind of doctor.

My decision had immediate repercussions. It was exhilarating to find out that if I just changed myself for the better, the rest of the world would somehow be forced to follow suit.

99

What happened that day was that I spoke out for more humane and sensitive patient care. The nurses constantly spoke out for all this, but the doctors didn't pay much attention to them. The actual issue focused on one of our patient's right to die in peace. You can imagine the taboo surrounding this topic.

To the medicine man death was natural and expected. Life and death were part of the rhythmic process of nature, and one passed on to the happy hunting ground whenever he was ripe and the spirit called.

In our strange medical culture, death meant 'Failure!' If you had a patient die in your service, that reflected terribly on you. It meant you were a bad doctor. The less death there was when you were on, the more impressive your record.

This whole approach reminded me of a game we used to play in summer camp called 'Jack's alive'. Somebody would hold a stick in the fire for a while until it was smoldering, and then take it out, smoky and hot. You could blow on the end and it would turn bright red with the heat from inside. You'd pass it to the next guy and say "Jack's alive", then he'd take it and blow on it and it would turn red. He'd pass it on and say "Jack's alive", and the stick would go around to everyone at the campfire. Then there would come a point which you couldn't see a red flame no matter how hard you blew. And you'd have to say "Jack's dead". The guy who had to say it got his face all smeared with black from the stick.

It was similar in the hospital. Death was always the enemy. It didn't matter if the patient were 80 years old, or 90 or 100. But it began to matter to me, so I spoke up. His name was Mr. Feli, an 86-year old Philippino man who was kept alive in a stupor for what could have been months (quite unnecessarily, it seemed to me). The medical staff just refused to let him go. He was constantly tortured by more and more diagnostic tests. He'd had a stroke, he had diabetes that was far advanced, and he had some sort of bowel obstruction. It was time for him to die, but they wouldn't let him go.

His regular doctor would be caring for him in the day time, but at night it would be whoever was on that night, and every night there would be a different doctor. If he died while you were on, then you had failed all the people who had been taking care of him for all these weeks. The main problem was that he was old and emaciated. He was never going to recover or even regain consciousness.

His aged wife would sometimes come to the hospital and try to talk to the doctors. I remember her saying to me in a very gentle voice, "You know, my husband used to tell me that when it came to be his time he hoped he would be able to die in peace." This lady was trying as diplomatically as possible to tell me to give her husband a chance to go more comfortably. He wasn't forty and having a mild heart attack, he was 86 and had spent his life. Now he probably wanted to be left alone.

One of the floor nurses, JoAnn Riggs, pulled me aside and asked, "Why don't you guys listen to her?" At that time in my career, I regret to say, I was not considering that I had to answer to the nurses. I had been trained that I knew best.

But it was getting more and more difficult to put in a new I.V. because most of his veins had been burned out already. It kept getting harder to find a new one so I had to dig deeper. He would scratch and squirm and sometimes moan. He was definitely suffering in his attempt to pass from his life. And we were keeping him alive, prolonging his pain. We even hooked him up to a respirator once or twice, and were constantly pushing drugs.

After he finally, at great length, died, we gathered for the clinical pathological conference. This is what we called the CPC, where all the doctors get together and talk over the case. We'd discuss what could have been done better, what went wrong, or what really happened. At CPC's the younger doctors would describe what they did and how they understood it. Then some wiser doctors would get up and explain how the 'youngsters' had totally blown it. Often the pathologist would make a diagnosis that had been completely overlooked. For instance, he might sometimes point to a severed aorta and say, "Here's what was really wrong. It was an aortic aneurism and not colon cancer at all."

At this particular CPC where we were discussing the old Philippino's death, all was in order without surprises. For the chief of medicine it was a routine case and everything was proper. He was ready to end the conference with his usual, "Are there any additional comments or questions?"

By then, my attitude had changed a bit. I recalled the wife, and the nurse, and the weeks of his moaning were still fresh in my mind. Here was my chance. I stood up before all the other doctors (interns, residents, attendings, and the chief of medicine) to speak my piece. My heart was painfully pounding. "I think we could have done better. I think we could have not strung this out so interminably. Why did we have to prolong this man's agony for weeks and weeks?"

There was a lot of buzzing on the part of the staff. But the chief, standing with erect and dignified composure, said very calmly and forcefully, "We did it to keep this man alive as long as possible."

That was not the point, not an answer at all, in my mind. My adrenalin was really flowing now. "But why," I pursued, "did we keep him alive for as long as possible? What was the point of doing that? He never would have recovered anyway, and he was really suffering."

There was a charge in the room you could touch. The chief took a deep breath, looked me in the eye, paused some more, and said in a slow condescending voice, "One of the things you are here to learn, Doctor, is good medicine. And sometimes at a teaching institution we will use cases like this one to teach you all the life-saving, life-preserving, and life-prolonging maneuvers that are possible. That's what's done at any good teaching institution, and that's what we were doing. We were teaching you the best possible medicine."

I felt my legs quavering slightly, and I knew my voice would do the same. I remembered Mr. Fitz, and the nurse who showed me that consciousness-raising was an important part of her work. I couldn't stop now.

"Wouldn't teaching us the best medicine mean doing for everybody all the time exactly what was most appropriate? Instead of prolonging this man's agony, we could learn when is an appropriate time to let go and when is not appropriate. Wouldn't that be learning the best possible medicine?"

This time the chief banged his fist on the table and almost shouted, "No, it wouldn't; not at this hospital. Sit down, Doctor."

I sat down, but the point was made. Everyone knew in his heart that prolonging agony for educational purposes was a somewhat seedy policy. Yet the chief was right when he said that any good teaching hospital does it. A good feeling came over me as I realized that my questions were like the group's repressed conscience speaking out.

103

As we filed out of the conference room, several of the younger doctors came up to me. They were genuinely appreciative that I had stuck my neck out to even touch on the issue of patient's rights and humane treatment. One, named Webster, wanted to talk in private. He was tall, smartly dressed, and had a beefy mid-west smile. A resident in his third year, he told me how two years ago an intern attempted suicide, but fortunately survived. Then, last year, an intern here had actually succeeded.

"Rich, it's amazing. I checked back over the records. Every year for the last five years at least one intern or resident at this hospital attempts to kill himself." He drew closer and searched my eyes internally. "You know, at big county hospitals they actually take an additional intern, just to replace the one they are liable to lose through suicide. It's just statistics to them."

I felt numb. Maybe I was this year's candidate.

The reason Webster had told me this story was that at a similar CPC meeting he, too, had risen to confront the chief. "What about this guy who committed suicide? I think that's something we should talk about, something that we as a profession need to deal with."

The chief had replied, "What! Are you accusing the people in this room of having anything at all to do with that? A troubled intern commits suicide over personal problems that began long before he worked here. Do you think that's something we have to discuss? Is that our fault?"

So he, too, had been told to sit down, and we immediately felt a connection. He wanted to know if anyone in my group was in danger.

"You mean, other than me?" We both laughed and went down

to the cafeteria for a cup of coffee and the start of a new friendship.

I didn't know it at the time, but there was an intern in big trouble. Larry Eggerly was so close to killing himself that I think he was saved only by a very astute nurse-counselor. Beth was talking to him one day and his voice sounded distant and strange. In fact, he was looking even more haggard than usual. She asked him if there was anything wrong. He replied, "No, no, no. I'm just very, very busy." But she detected something in his tone, and convinced him to go with her to a quiet place and talk. Beth was older, well-trained, and a very good listener.

The other nurses were giving him a hard time. He wasn't doing everything he was supposed to, and the doctors weren't giving him any support whatsoever. He was just finding it more and more overwhelming, more and more difficult, and he began to think that maybe it was somehow all his fault. His nerves were shot from lack of sleep. Eggerly had arrived thinking he was pretty capable, a good scientist and a good student. All of this was true. But now they were telling him he was slow and that he didn't know his right hand from his left when it came to learning the drugs and procedures. His case presentations were a mess. In fact, his whole dream of being a doctor was collapsing in a welter of inadequacy, and he had nothing left. Without Beth's sensitive listening he might have been the Suicide of the Year. She advised that he take a vacation, and he came back restored.

I realized how similar my own feelings had been to Eggerly's, and possibly to the intern in the year ahead of me who succeeded in killing himself. Webster told me that he did it in a very unusual way. He took one of those long intracardiac needles and drew up a cocktail of many different drugs into a big syringe. Then he took the long cardiac needle at the end of the syringe, stuck it into his own heart, and pumped the drug into the needle. It was very Japanese, a medical hari-kari that was extremely effective.

It's interesting that he chose the heart. Heart disease was once called the 'doctor's illness', because so many doctors have heart attacks. It was getting easy to see how a sensitive young doctor might get a broken heart and how an insensitive older doctor might get a clogged heart.

I was really shaken up by Webster's story. Somehow, in addition to being hazardous to patients, the medical system was hazardous to the health of doctors. It was not hard to see how true this was for interns. That one year was a terribly frenzied time, where we were constantly told that we were no good, and that we weren't worth anything. We ate our food on the run, often out of vending machines, with no chance to digest whatever questionable nourishment there was. These machines supplied us health-givers with cardboard, phlegmy, chemical-flavored stews and pieces of soggy, sugar-filled dough called pastry. Overdoses of caffeine prevented our collapse.

The chief of medicine, for example, had a perpetual cigarette going in one hand and a cup of coffee in the other. It's hard to see how he ever held a stethescope. He would light a new cigarette with the previous one. He later had his heart attack at age forty-four. And there he was trying to take care of everyone else, training young doctors to be more like him, to make the world a healthier place.

On checking a few articles in the hospital library, I found that in addition to heart disease and suicide, doctors have much higher rates of divorce and drug addiction than the general population. When I saw how hazardous this whole scene was to my own health, and how in a very graphic way that made it hazardous to the health of someone like Jay Fitz, I became still more driven to do something.

I hated to admit it at the time, but one of the compensations for me was just the same thing for which I was angry at the chief - Power. I sure got off on my own sense of authority, the power that came with the magical new title of 'doctor'.

I am not an imposing physical presence. In fact I am rather short and almost skinny. So I got real pleasure when often hefty men would come under my jurisdiction and let me order them around. It took me a while to get used to the fact that I could get them to do anything I wanted. I shared something with generals, dictators, or orchestra conductors, and revelled in it for a while.

For instance, one of my first cases was a six foot eight, two hundred fifty pound guy, rough and mean looking. It would have scared me to talk to him out on the street even in broad daylight. As part of every physical you're supposed to do a rectal exam. So when the time came, somewhat to my surprise he meekly lay sideways on the table, and at my bidding put his knee up, and held still while I stuck my finger up his rectum. If he told me it was hurting I could tell him, "Too bad, I know it hurts, but this is what I have to do." And if he told me he didn't want me to draw blood, I would tell him that he was required to cooperate. What power! I guess the chief was doing the same thing to us in a different way.

To make up for having power I sometimes had to put up with terrible smells. I'll never forget the odor of the emergency room. First there would be the blood, usually from a patient getting hit over the head with a bottle or a billy club. Then there was the booze, and one could tell if it was beer, wine, or hard liquor. And I musn't leave out the vomit, either fresh from recent hot dogs or old and stale. This

107

unique mixture was the most awful stench imaginable. It was the stench of decay, from the unhappiest and most unfortunate elements of our society. I never really got used to it.

This odor was filling my lungs two nights later while I was working on the muscular hulk of a young black man. He was drunk and vomiting, and I'd had a terrible time quieting him enough so that he'd lie down. I had to talk for quite a while with just the right mixture of gentleness and firmness, so that he was finally beginning to let me sew up a deep skull laceration which was gushing blood. I was fairly new to the procedure, and it was slow going.

Just then Frank Saxby came by. A fellow intern, Frank seemed to me especially insensitive and somewhat of a jerk. Nevertheless he'd just finished his surgery rotation, so he knew a bit more about sewing than I did. Spying his chance to show me a thing or two, he came over just as the patient finished another bout of vomiting and then had lain back, seemingly unconscious.

"How'd this dummy get cut so deep?" Frank asked nonchalantly. All of a sudden the 'unconscious' patient sat up with amazing speed, and said in an ominous bass tone, "You in trouble, boy."

It was quite a sight. Frank knew he was in trouble and blurted out, "OK, I'm going, you don't have to worry."

It didn't matter. The massive, angry black man lurched up and started going after Frank, blood dripping out of his head, two I.V. bottles dragging on the floor, held in by tubes that were taped to his arms. His white gown was dragging strings, so that he was tripping all over himself, which increased his rage. Slowed by drunkenness and loss of blood, he came within a foot of Frank, who barely escaped through the door with his life.

108

Patients always sense and hear what's going on at some level, even when they are under anesthesia. They pick up readily on the attitude of the staff towards them. They can tell whether they are thought of as a piece of meat or as a human being. With those on the bottom rungs of the social ladder, it's too frequently the former, and it saddens me every time I see it.

Too many things were wrong and needed upgrading. They were pent up in each of us, festering. Non-communication was everywhere - barriers between staff and patients, between doctors and nurses, and even among the interns themselves. Not being able to share our true feelings with each other made it almost unbearable for some of us. The time had come to do something different.

A few days later, several of us were standing around outside the operating room discussing the CPC, the E.R. chase scene, and intern suicides. Discontent hung heavy, but was leading nowhere. Vague mumblings had occasionally been heard about some sort of internship group. Finally I said, "Look, here are three of us who've been bitching fruitlessly for months and nothing ever happens. I hear that Bella, the surg nurse, has a consciousness-raising group with nurses. Why don't we, right now, form our own group? We could talk over our feelings and plan some changes."

That next day the hospital P.A. system startled quite a few people when it carried this announcement: "The first meeting of the Internship Association will be tonight at the home of Dr. Richard Shames." The hospital operator and pager was our friend so we had her repeat it a few times.

It had major political impact. Now the Internship Association was a reality, and we had to be taken more seriously. But what felt even more important was the chance for us all to get together as a group and talk about what was happening.

We were actually an internship support group, arising from the need to share our feelings about literally life and death matters. We discussed issues such as my thoughts about Mr. Fitz, or Eggerly's near suicide or how we felt about hopeless cases or the way the residents were putting us down. We met once a week, and it was a fundamental change. Later in the year, we even invited a few of the nurses to come share with us.

Many of us had believed that our feelings of inadequacy were somewhat unique. At the meeting, it slowly dawned on us that others were having the same problems, and had been going through similar emotions. This made our own individual situations a whole lot easier to bear.

The knowledge that we now had each other for support was enough to change our attitudes and sense of power. From out of this change, our lives began to work more smoothly and with greater health. I learned a great deal that year.

I'll never forget that whole long series of special patients. I remain appreciative for the older doctors who taught me diagnosis and treatment. But I especially remember the sensitivity and dedication of the nurses.

Of course there was Bella, who gave us the idea of forming a group. Eggerly is especially grateful to Beth, who saved him from becoming the 'Intern of the Year'. But there were a great many more whose firm conviction on the art of healing laid a strong foundation, and inspired me to become a better doctor.

For instance, when I once asked Jennifer to help me draw some blood for repeat cultures that I needed right now, she said, "Sure, as

110

soon as I finish this backrub." I remember being livid! How could she waste precious time like that when there were crucial things to be done - like repeating the blood cultures. Now, as I see things more clearly, what she was doing was probably much more therapeutic than what I was doing - and she knew it.

Marguerite, a charge nurse on the Pulmonary Service, unknowingly taught me the value of holding the hand of bedridden patients whenever telling them something very important.

My pelvic exams became quite a bit more humane when Lucille helped me out one day. A plump and sassy OB L.P.N., she told the patient to try to relax and not to blame the doctor if it hurt, because "he's just busy and gotta go fast". I realized that not hurting her had to become a priority for me - how could I unconsciously inflict pain on people who were coming to me with pain? It just didn't make sense.

Even more direct was Cathy, from the Rehab Department. She always made what I then thought was the useless effort of pleasantly talking to stroke or accident victims who seemed totally 'out to lunch'. One day between doing stomach tubes, I quickly sandwiched in a suturing job on one of her patients. She stopped me in the hall immediately afterwards with a clear, strong, and neutral voice. "Next time you have a painful procedure to do, the patient and I would appreciate your using some anesthetic." Knowing she was right, I mumbled "OK", and walked off. Even as I turned, I realized I should have added, "and thank you, nurse".

Many other docs may not have thanked her. Maybe they would have yelled at her and put her in her place. But I knew she was right, and those other docs were not my role models anymore.

I now felt a lot better about Mr. Fitz, Mr. Feli, and about myself. A new entity was beginning to emerge: a more sensitive kind of doctor; a good listener as well as a good diagnostician; a more open-minded team player; and a more compassionate healer.

Postscript

Now, more than twenty years have passed since that early intern-ship disenchantment. The medicine man images led me to explore hypnosis, herbal remedies, acupuncture, homeopathy, yoga, vitamin therapy, and biofeedback, among other tools. I do my expanded brand of general medicine in parallel practice with my wife, Karilee (an R.N. who offers counseling, preventive care, dance therapy, and bodywork).

I feel blessed to have had this extra growth and development. I especially urge my medical colleagues to keep an open mind and open heart in regard to nursing's empowerment. These developments can only serve to elevate the quality of health care for us all.

And, to the nurses, I offer my deeply felt gratitude, and my highest hopes for your collective success. (Start more and more of your own support groups, and may the 'nurse' be with you!)

113

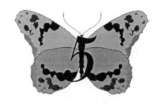

EMERGING FROM THE
WHITE COCOON
One Nurse's
'Shocking' Revelation

NOTE: Every nurse has a story to tell, and this is part of mine. I share it in the spirit of removing our masks, uncovering our wounds, and inspiring collective healing through telling our truths. If this inspires you to write your own story, you may feel lighter and freer from the experience. Part of my dream is to create a future book dedicated solely to our stories, so feel free to send yours on to me. This represents my early search into the heart - and soul - of nursing.

Karilee Halo Shames, R.N., Ph.D. is a writer, lecturer, dancer, and devoted mother of two daughters and a son. She received her B.S. Nursing, B.A. Sociology, and M.S. Nursing at the University of Maryland, as well as a special training at Walter Reed Army Medical Center.

She pursued graduate level education in alternative universities.

In 1977, she co-founded a national nurses' support network, and now maintains a private practice in nurse counseling and women's issues. In 1987 she created Nurse Empowerment Workshops & Services (NEWS), a motivational and consulting firm which offers morale-building hospital presentations and specializes in team-building for dysfunctional units. She also presents a series of off-site healing seminars (The Nightingale Conspiracy Retreats).

"Hello, Pearl. I'm Karilee. I'll be helping to take care of you today."

"Papa peed, and Mama peed . . . Papa peed, and Mama peed . . ." she answered.

What in the world? Could I believe my ears? I looked down at the tiny figure stuffed in amongst the bed pillows. As I contemplated the meaning of her message, her roommate spoke up.

"She's blind as a bat. Can't even see light."

That changed things for me. Poor Pearl . . . living alone in a dark dream world, perched on that chair, belting out a song as the sparrow sings, calling out to the world in ways that man cannot comprehend. I gave up my search to find meaning in her words, and looked at her name band.

"Pearl White. February 11, 1862." How appropriate, the name. She was a perfect person to wear the name Pearl White if ever I met one. As I pondered that, another thought bombarded my brain. "1862! Why, that was the last century!".

"That's right," her roommate, Milly, read my mind. "She's 103 years old."

I stared at Pearl, with her pearly white skin and hair. Never had I met anyone so old. The picture of her, propped up among those pillows, touched my most tender place. Here was history, right in a small body in Memorial Hospital, Room 216.

"Papa peed, and Mama peed . . . Papa peed, and Mama peed . . ."

I was thirteen years old, and this was my first week as a candystriper (volunteer) at Memorial Hospital. I felt flushed and full of excitement as I scrutinized the person responsible for that tiny, silly song.

Her hair was white, and fell in fine wisps around her face and down her back. Her face was thin, with folds of skin where cheeks had once been full. I could even see faint white eyelashes, as I moved closer, lashes that encircled large green eyes that focused in one direction, carrying a far-away look within.

Her roommate, Milly, offered more data. "She sings those words day and night, day in and day out." Though Milly tried to appear irritated, I could tell that Pearl had won a soft spot in her heart nonetheless, as she was soon to do to mine. "She'll stop it, though, soon as you talk to her."

Suddenly, as if to honor our conservation, the chanting stopped. I sat down on a straight chair next to her, and took her tiny, birdlike hand in mine. I spoke loud and slowly.

"Pearl, I am Karilee. Do you hear me?"

"Yes. I am Karilee too. Do you hear me?"

I burst out laughing, then quickly covered my mouth. I certainly didn't want to show any disrespect to someone who had been alive eight times as long as I had!

We spent hours talking, Pearl and I, as days melted into weeks,

117

making us both old-timers in that place. Pearl was the one patient I came to consider 'my first great love'. It turned out that she may have been blind, but her mind was sharp as could be, and she was never at a loss for something to say.

I asked her many things, and she always came back quickly with something that sounded reasonable, yet hit my funny bone at the same time. Soon, my nights at home were devoted to thinking up things to ask Pearl. I asked her about fashions, customs, and events from days of yore.

One night I came up with the ultimate question, and there was no sleep for the weary that night, so great was my anticipation. What would she say? Would it be true? How could I tell?

The next afternoon, I raced breathlessly into Room 16.

There she was, my friend Pearl, chanting as usual. "Papa peed, and mama peed.. Papa peed and Mama peed . . ."

"Pearl. PEARL . . . This is Karilee.

"This is Karilee . . . Papa peed and Mama peed . . ."

"Pearl. I have something I want to ask you, and it's very important that you tell me the truth."

"What is it? Tell me the truth."

I knew she was with me then, so I proceeded.

"Pearl, your chart says you were a nurse during the Crimean War.§ Is that true?"

---

§ It was not until some years later that I learned that, despite her advanced age, Pearl could not have been a nurse in the Crimean War. The Crimean War ended in 1856!

118

"Yes, I was a nurse."

"Do you remember how to make hospital corners?" I added this to test her out. Maybe she was leading me on?

"Of course I can make hospital corners. I made thousands of beds in my day."

"How do you do it?" I asked, curious to see what she would say.

"Why, you take the corner part of the top sheet, turn it under the mattress . . ." she drifted off.

"Then what, Pearl? What do you do to the sheet then?"

"You turn it under the mattress . . . then cut it with some scissors."

I laughed out loud. She laughed too.

"Pearl, did you know Florence Nightingale?"

This time I watched her very carefully for any giveaway signs. She looked like she was searching way back in memory.

"Yes, of course I knew her. I knew Florence Nightingale."

Breathlessly I whispered, "What was she like?"

"What was who like?" she asked.

"Florence Nightingale, Pearl. What kind of person was she?"

Her voice came loud and strong. "She was the biggest darn whore there ever was."

All my hopes, dashed in one small sentence. No, I'll never forget Pearl.

~   ~   ~   ~   ~

It's not easy to tell you why I became a nurse. I can only say

119

that my need to be a nurse was etched on my soul as surely as the freckles on my face. For me, the pull was like a plant growing toward the light, a bird flying south for winter, or a nun hearing her calling.

That's even the more reason why my disillusionment with nursing shocked me; it made a liar of my soul. How could I need to be a nurse, and at the same time, feel so strongly that what I was doing was wrong?

To me, a nurse can be a minister of healing. As with other ministries, the adversity must be used to inspire one to try harder; to reach greater heights. Maybe this will help you understand why I am one of those nurses who will always be a nurse, no matter where I am or what else I am doing.

Maybe I was *born* a nurse . . . My father says I always wanted to be one. I don't remember that as clearly as I recall the endless hours spent with friends exploring each others' bodies, playing the eternal game of 'doctor'.

My real professional history, however, started at the age of thirteen. Suddenly, amidst raging adolescent hormones, I woke up one day with a burning desire to do my healing work. I called the local hospital and inquired about candystriping possibilities. They asked if I was fourteen.

"Oh, yes," I replied breathlessly, regretting instantly the decision to lie, but absolutely certain that nothing was to get in the way of my budding aspirations. It was more important to get inside those hospital walls at that moment than anything else in the world, and I knew I would be absolved.

I donned the red and white striped uniform I had purchased

with glowing pride. I had indeed become someone very important overnight. After attending the orientation program at Memorial Hospital, I was turned loose in the endless corridors, loving every precious minute I spent there.

To me, the hospital was filled with great intrigue. It was a magnificent world unto itself, not unlike Camelot might have appeared to a young, impressionable Arthur. At each turn, my nose was greeted with another strange and curious odor. In every direction, I could hear the pitter-patter of soft shoes racing against shined linoleum floors. The fast pace conveyed a constant sense of urgency, increasing my belief that I was intimately involved in a brave and heroic mission.

On weekends, while my family piled into our old Caddy and drove to the beach for handball and swimming, I begged to be dropped off at Memorial. Certainly there were more important things to do than just sit around absorbing the Florida rays.

At that point in my life, excitement came from carrying lovely floral arrangements into hospital rooms, and reading the neatly written notes to grateful people propped in hospital beds. They seemed thirsty for the good wishes behind each gift. Sometimes I would delay for a moment to talk further with the lucky recipient of the flowers, and even to try to be sensitive to the person in the next bed who might not have been so lucky.

Whenever I entered a room, I took it upon myself to brighten it up somehow, and to leave its occupants more comfortably nestled in their beds, with pillows fluffed and water pitchers full. Most often, I got to sit for a minute while the patient told me all about so-and-so, who had sent the thoughtful flowers.

121

It always surprised me how these small acts could perk up even the grayest-looking face, and somewhere along the line I decided that even more than the gift, *the act of feeling and expressing love was a crucial factor in healing.* I vowed to store this bit of information in my brain for future reference, for even then I was certain that my simple actions had actually been a form of gentle medicine.

On my sixteenth birthday, my parents gave the ultimate gift - my very own car! She was a beauty, ol' Bessie, a turquoise and white '59 Chevy, complete with the big wings and cats eye lights in back. I loved it, and though it had cost only $350, I felt like a millionaire.

It wasn't long, however, before I discovered that Bessie had an insatiable appetite. Once again, I found myself seeking work in health care. This time, though, it was different. This time, I had to be paid for it, and instead of a hospital, I tried my luck at a nursing home.

I was dauntless. When they asked if I had any experience, my answer was boldly positive. "Sure, I've had plenty of experience. I worked at Memorial for years." I didn't expand on that enough to inform them that my work there had been strictly volunteer.

"O.K.," the voice on the line said. "Good thing you called. We happen to be in a real bind today. Can you be here at 2:30? You'll work till eleven, it pays $1.10 an hour, and you need a uniform. You'll be temporary until your interview."

The phone dropped back onto its cradle from my trembling fingers. "Oh, my God! Now what am I going to do?" I screamed, as I tore across the room in search of the uniform I didn't own. "2:30 today, and I don't have a uniform, shoes, or nylons . . . what in the

122

world was I thinking?"

My voice trailed off into an eerie silence as I tried to regain my composure. It was already noon, and I had to figure out where this place was. Panic clutched at my heart, and I then figured out what to do, and felt calm.

Two hours later, with great embarrassment, I stuck my head in the front door of Collier Manor Nursing Home, painfully conscious of my candy-cane garb. "It's O.K., girl, it's alright . . ." I soothed myself just as I would my patients. Time after time in later years, this ability would come in very handy, especially when I had bitten off more than I could comfortably chew.

After the briefest of orientations, I was still scared to death. Someone handed me a list of room numbers and mumbled something about the lady in room 21A with a lift (did she say "lisp"?), and to watch the man in 23C (or did she say "watch out for him?").

"Excuse me," I bravely stuttered. "This is my first day here and I didn't hear what you said." As I looked up, my panic was overshadowed by the irony of the situation. No one had heard what I said either. There I was alone, in a urine-scented corridor.

My fright began to melt into curiosity as I searched above the doorways for one of those numbers. "18, 20, 22, . . . where are the odd numbers?" "Oops — sorry!" I gasped as I ran into someone in the hall.

"Odd numbers are on the other side of the nurse's station. Who are you trying to find?" I looked into the kind eyes of a janitor, an old fellow who could easily have spent every waking minute of the last fifty years pushing that broom down this hall. I glanced at my list again.

"Mr. Jackley. Room 23C." I tried out my most confident voice.

Suddenly he burst out laughing. "Wha-a-at? They gave him to you?" He held onto his broom handle and laughed right from his wide belly. "Lady, this must not be your lucky day." I could hear him chuckling way down the hall as he turned to go. I felt my courage beginning to droop and sag around my ankles. Quickly, I picked myself up and stomped past the nurses' station, where I drew more than one look from the staff.

I marched, attempting to look fearless, into room 23C. After all, I knew what I was here for, and by jove, I was going to do a great job! Suddenly, though, my feet stood still, and I felt frozen to that spot. I held my breath as his eyes met mine. There he was, the patient in bed 23C, and he did look wild. His name tag said Lionel Jackley, and he had a stump for a leg, and eyes that crossed as if he were looking beyond you.

"NURSE! NURSE! COME HELP ME!" He was tied to his bed with the side rails up, and I was reminded of a trapped animal I once watched, struggling to free itself from captivity. The strangest part of witnessing this scene, though, was noticing how I felt. Suddenly I felt trapped as well! What could be the matter with him? Why were they treating him like this? The questions danced through my brain as I backed out the door. "I'm sorry, Mr. Jackley," I heard myself mumbling as I once again marched to the nurses' station.

This time I planted my feet firmly on the ground and demanded an answer. When someone finally looked at me, I managed to latch on to her eyes with all my intent focused into that stare, and as our eyes locked, I spoke. "What is the matter with Mr. Jackley, and why is he tied up like that?" She seemed to flush, almost imperceptibly, then began to ramble off a list of medical terms.

124

"I don't understand. Please, tell me in simple English, so I know how to care for him." Seldom do I remember being so clear, and so bold. To my delight, it paid off then. She sighed emphatically, as if to indicate that she had better things to do, then told me that his brain wasn't working clearly anymore, that he had lost his leg recently from diabetes infection, and that no one seemed to care enough to visit him, as he had been here a while with no inquiries or guests. Her response to my question as to how to care for him came in one word: "quickly".

With that, I turned and headed for 23C. When I got there, I paused outside, silently mustering up the courage to re-enter his room. I heard footsteps softly approaching behind me, and I spun around on my heel. I was face-to-face with a gentle-looking woman, probably close to 50 years old, with deep black eyes that were surrounded by many smile wrinkles, and her short curly red hair.

She was smaller than my 5'1" frame, and the name tag on her uniform read 'Mercedes More, N.A.'. So, finally, here was someone in my lowly category, another Nurses Aide. Maybe she could make sense of some of this. When she spoke, she looked young, with a sparkle in her eyes and a song in her voice. Her words came slowly, through broken English.

"He ees not crasee. He ees, how do you say, confoosed? I talk to heem every day. He ees muy lonely." I smiled at her attempt to sound American with such a strong Cuban accent, and knew instantly that we would get along real well. Fortunately, I could speak Spanish, and when Mercedes realized this, she danced with joy.

I found out everything I could about Mr. Jackley. He had no family, and Room 23, Bed C was destined to be his last stop in life. The nurses seemed to have no time or patience for him, so they would either slam the door on him, or increase his tranquilizers. It made me wonder what had changed his supposedly-tender caregivers into nurses who seemed unaffected by his dismal plight.

His bed was indeed his cage, and you could hear his side rails rattle into the night. They had given him a 'pet name' (how appropriate), and referred to him as 'Mad Dog Jackley'. I began to wonder which had come first, his treatment or his wild behavior. Perhaps his bizarre actions were an appropriate response to his situation.

I was determined to become more familiar with him, and thus began to spend as much time as I could visiting him. Little by little, I allowed some slack in his arm restraints. It was such a small gift, that tiny bit of freedom to move. Just when I was indulging in some righteous indignation about the whole situation, a strange thing happened.

I had pulled the thermometer out from between the folds of his buttocks (they told me not to take his temperature orally, in case he should bite down). I turned around to record his temp on the chart, when I felt the slightest rustle in the back of my uniform. Before I had a chance to respond, I saw that he had reached out from the bed and put his hand up my skirt.

I felt a hot flush rising, and imagined how odd I must look with my redness screaming out against a red and white dress. My mind felt jumbled; my thoughts rambled in various directions. If I let him continue, would I regret it? Would I be sorry if I didn't?

That last thought shocked me - yet, there I was sixteen, and wanting to save the world. My stubborn attitude had gotten me into this - how would I ever get out?

For a fleeting moment, I wondered if he was responding to

126

something I had done. After all, I had invaded his personal and intimate space with my procedures; maybe this was his response. On the other hand, maybe his brain was working better than any of us knew, and he had conjured up a way to make me feel the way he felt. I knew that human bodies crave touch, much as plants thirst for water. Yet, I had been told to avoid him; "He's just a crazy old man".

What was crazy? He was right; he did need help. But, was this the way to ask for it? Would he see my negative reaction as another rejection? How could I best help him?

My picture of what I should have done went like this: I'd remove his hand from beneath my uniform and hold it. "I like you, Mr. Jackley," I'd begin, "and I'd like to get to know you better. I'm sure it's not fun being tied to that bed, and maybe we can figure out a way to make things more comfortable and pleasant."

What actually happened, however, was different than that. To be truthful, his touch felt good. I knew this wasn't an unhealthy thing for a man to do, nor was it unhealthy for me to feel turned on. What was unhealthy was the situation . . . all of it! What did Florence Nightingale do at times like this?

I really don't know what she would have done (was Pearl really right?), but I let Mr. Jackley have a minute or two of harmless touch. That experience has been with me ever since.

~   ~   ~   ~   ~

It was also here that I encountered Mrs. Fish, the lady with the lift (it wasn't lisp). When I first walked into her room and inhaled, it occurred to me that they called her that because of the odor. It turned out, however, that it really was her name. She weighed close to 300 pounds and the lift was a piece of machinery, similar to a crane, used to turn her from side to side. She was unable to control her bowel or bladder, so one needed to use the lift frequently to change her sheets.

That poor woman was as difficult as Mr. Jackley, but in a different way. She was blind, soiled her sheets at regular intervals during the day and night, and had to be fed baby food because she had no teeth. They weren't kidding when they said they were in a bind that afternoon - it turned out there was only one nurse and one aide to work with me. Together, we were responsible for covering a wing with twenty-two patients on it.

Standing alone in Mrs. Fish's room, I looked at the scene before me and prayed for help. I didn't want to appear stupid or pesty, but I couldn't fathom how to move that enormous body, and frankly, just the thought of it made me queasy. Each time I tried to roll her to one side, thinking I could somehow move the sheet over to one side, then out, my fingers slid from the perspiration on her skin.

Again and again I made futile efforts to extract the ammonia-smelling sheet, until eventually, whenever I pushed against the folds in her thighs, I gagged. How would I ever get her cleaned up - and deep within my private thoughts bobbed an even less acceptable question - why? I muddled my way through till eleven, after someone showed me how to change her, then finally went home. I jumped into a hot, soapy bath, followed by a shower.

The next day was my formal interview, and I was tingling with excitement. The Director of Nursing, Miss Pearlocker, gave me an orientation, explained the set-up, and described the type of patients housed in this facility. I now felt much better about Collier Manor, and was formally hired for the 3-11 shift.

Despite her metal glasses and military stance, Miss Pearlocker had a heart of gold, and I felt warmth from her. I looked forward to each day at Collier Manor, and knew I was learning a lot there, not only about patient care, but about the politics of health care as well. For example, I discovered that the patients who were private, paying customers were treated quite differently than those receiving government subsidy.

Since many of the patients were bed-ridden, the nurses' aides had to turn them regularly to prevent bedsores from forming. Unfortunately, a large percentage of these people had already acquired those ghastly craters, which looked exactly like volcanic openings in the skin. The private patients were treated with many fancy preparations, ones which cleaned the dead skin out, then cleansing solutions, topped by sterile gauze pads covered with expensive cortisone creams. Often, prior to the bandages being applied, the skin ulcer was cleansed and exposed to special lights to kill bacteria and dry out the wounds.

Meanwhile, in another room down the hall, a patient with bedsores was also receiving treatment; this time, the aid would pull off the old bandage, pour in some hydrogen peroxide, and after wiping out the frothing liquid, pour in some brown sugar! I could hardly believe my eyes when I first witnessed that. "Why brown sugar?", I asked, as another aide demonstrated the procedure. "Because," she answered in a monotone, "this is the poor folks' cortisone. The bacteria likes to eat on it."

As times passed, I became more comfortable and familiar with procedures such as this. Occasionally, I asked to change jobs with the Licensed Vocational Nurse, Miss Brown. Though it was not an easy or pleasant position, her job had some distinct advantages. She walked from room to room, pushing a little treatment cart. The patients knew her as 'the treatment nurse', and many patients groaned when they heard the squeaky wheels approaching their room.

Miss Brown taught me how to wash ulcerated feet and bodies, apply heat lamps to mutilated skin, and also to use this precious, though painful, time of contact to "wake up de doc inside", as she would say. She explained that she did this work as a result of having been severely injured in a car accident years ago. She prayed at that time to be made whole again, and said that Jesus came to her in a dream, and told her he would heal her, and then wanted her to go around helping other people to heal. She said that Jesus told her there was a doctor inside every person, one who knows how to heal that special person. Her job was to wake people up to that inner healer. (I was later to read something quite similar by Albert Schweitzer).

This was very challenging work for me. Since I did not come from a strong religious background that provided me with such a deep well of faith, I often found myself asking why I was doing such disgusting things to people. There were several times when I felt that I couldn't cope.

Occasionally, I would peer into the debrided ulcer after the dead cells had been cleaned out. When I'd look inside the area, surrounded by shiny red flesh, I could see bones where there was no flesh left. I wondered why their insides didn't spill out onto the bed; I also wondered what it was like for them to live through this slow, tortuous demise.

Once, when I asked an old man about that, his cynical answer hit me deep in my gut. He said he felt like a prisoner with no trial, no parole, and no release in sight. I came to understand that it was not these slow, chronic problems that caused their decline. Ultimately, it seemed to be their attitude that mattered above all else.

130

I could see how their susceptibility to more fatal conditions increased as the will to live diminished. Just as many prisoners kill themselves rather than live out their sentences, so did many of these persons create the illness that set them free. I learned that for some people, death is considered the ultimate cure; the final stage of healing, when the will to live has departed.

Thus, I grew to appreciate the dire importance of being a compassionate caregiver. Those precious, tender moments caring for a withered body allowed me a very privileged, gentle entry into the soul. Though I never really enjoyed the physical work, I lived for the union it created between me and my patient. My goal became to inspire, to share tenderness, and to help instill a will to live, or to surrender to the call of death peacefully, if that was most appropriate. In my highest vision, this is what nursing was all about.

And there I was, armed with my high ideals, when I first encountered a real nurse. Most of the people I had worked closely with were Nurses Aides, occasionally Licensed Practical Nurses. Miss Warner was different. She was a Registered Nurse, but even more, she was the charge nurse on B Wing.

Miss Susan Warner was a tiny young woman, less than five feet tall, with a small button nose and enormous brown eyes. Her hair was short, very bushy, and I thought she looked so wonderful in her sparkling white uniform. In an embarrassingly adolescent way, I developed a kind of 'school-girl' crush on her, and followed her around doing anything I could to help.

I managed to get assigned to her wing as often as possible, and my heart would sing as I drove Bessie in to begin work. Sometimes my mind would conjure up images of her with a man (surely there was some handsome man in her life), and I'd wonder what she did

131

when she wasn't at the nursing home.

At that stage of my life, everything seemed so glamorous and romantic, and I existed in a fantasy world much of the time. After many hours spent with her, I really didn't know much more about Miss Warner than I did initially. She didn't talk about herself much, certainly not to me.

That's why I was even more shocked and surprised one day when, after being assigned to an extra shift, I was coming through a folding door and encountered her - literally. We banged into each other, and I smiled in an awkward, goofy way, while she turned on me: "How come you're here so much? Don't you have anything better to do with your time? You must be a glutton for punishment." And she said it like she meant it.

"Glutton for punishment . . . glutton for punishment . . ." Those words reeled through my confused brain for hours after that. My dream world was shattered. What did she mean, "Glutton for punishment?".

Late that same night, in the dark comfort of my bed, I reflected on the events of the day. Miss Warner had seemed like one of the nicest nurses I could imagine. Did she really mean what she said? What was punishment? Maybe there was more to her job than I had known. Maybe she existed under pressures that my naive brain couldn't fathom. Many of the nurses I'd met there did seem brusque; perhaps angry.

Had they ever felt the tingling I felt when I was helping people? If so, what had happened? That experience with Miss Warner, more than anything else, engraved upon my heart a burning desire to explore the roots of nursing's anguish. Maybe there was more than

132

meets the eye?

After all, my sixth sense has always been one of my greatest strengths . . . It may have alerted me, then and there, to a level of frustration that surpassed Miss Warner, one that is perhaps nursing's deepest sorrow. I wondered if I would ever confront it myself, and vowed - if so - to get to the other side.

The following summer, and during the nursing school year as well, I worked part-time on an inpatient psychiatric unit. By then, I was much more aware of what I liked and didn't like in caring for people. I really liked the humane, caring part; and did not enjoy the technical aspects. I figured I owed it to myself to try mental health work.

This particular unit was in a small, religious affiliated hospital in the suburbs. I once again donned my uniform, having long ago invested in some nice white ones to replace my faithful candystriper one. As I entered for my first orientation, I received more than one odd stare. When the instructor began to talk to the handful of us assembled, the first thing she announced was that the staff on this unit wore street clothes. I felt silly in my uniform, though happy to hear the news. "It's about time," I thought, "that we relate more as regular people. What a smart idea!"

At the time, it was an innovative plan, an attempt to minimize trauma due to the association of white garb with 'those other nurses'. We were different; you could trust and count on us (or so I thought!).

The patients on this unit were awakened early, in order to allow for preparations and procedures prior to breakfast. I was surprised at the number of injections which were prepared and quickly administered at that early hour. "These are given prior to E.C.T." one nurse

133

told me. "It calms them".

"What's E.C.T.?", I bravely asked, when it became apparent that no one else would.

"Electro-Convulsive Therapy. Commonly referred to as Electroshock. It's one of our major forms of therapeutic intervention here."

Boy, was I shocked! I had heard about lobotomies, and other techniques that seemed to be remnants from a distant dark age; I just had no idea that electroshock was still used, much less on a unit where I would work.

I recalled touring Memorial Hospital years ago. As they marched us quickly through the locked part of the psychiatry unit, there was a small E.C.T. machine kept in a back room. "We don't use it much," I recall the head nurse saying, "It's only indicated for some very severe depressions when nothing else seems to help, kind of a last resort."

These words were ringing in my ears, and suddenly I felt chills running down my spine. "You can just get acquainted with the unit today," the instructor's voice trailed off as she bustled about, "and tomorrow they'll orient you on the procedure. Right now we'll serve breakfast trays to the patients as they return from their therapy. You can find out who they are from their name bands."

From their name bands? These people must be crazier than I imagined. Couldn't they even remember who they were? I was soon to discover how confused they were; more alarming, however, was to discover the cause of their confusion.

A lady came towards me in the hall. She was whimpering, and stumbling as her arm reached out to clutch my sweater. "Help me, help me," she mumbled, saliva rolling down her chin. I looked into her eyes, the window to her soul, but there was no one home. Vacant.

"I'll try." I said calmly. "What can I do?". She met my gaze with a hollow stare, as if she were looking through me, off into the distance.

"I need to call my daughter. She'll help me. I have to get out of here or they'll kill me for sure."

"Who are you?" I asked, just as one of the regular staff came around the corner.

"That's Mrs. Schiff," the aide said curtly. "She's ready for breakfast now."

"No, no . . ." the lady protested in a wavering voice. "I have to call my daughter. Please help me."

I looked searchingly at the nurses' aide, who proceeded to hustle about as if no one was there. "Ignore her," she said. "They're not allowed to make phone calls after shock."

"Why not?", I ventured.

"Because," she stated evenly, "they're too confused."

Mrs. Schiff did indeed seem confused, though not much more than I. "How does that happen?", I asked.

"Dunno, it just does."

As I glanced down the hall, I witnessed a very strange sight. A steady stream of vacant-looking bodies were being escorted by two men who I later found out were E.C.T. Aides. It was like a science fiction movie, and could have been an eerie parade of extraterrestrial beings. Some were crying, and several asked for aspirin as they clutched their head. The sight would have astounded even the most disinterested observer.

"I want to call my mother. I'm calling my mother right now." I turned to face a bewildered-looking girl, perhaps in her late teens, with red eyes and a very determined voice. "If you don't let me use the phone, I'm going to report it to the judge. They'll get you, you know."

Something felt very wrong here. I had looked towards psychiatry as a benign way of helping people, yet here it felt like staff and patients were on opposing teams.

"You can't do this to me," the young woman whimpered. "I have some rights, don't I?" She looked up at me.

"I don't know," I replied sullenly. "I'm sure you must." Her arm band said that she was Ellen Smith, and belonged in Room 14.

Ellen insisted that she belonged at home, but her mother threatened her with hospitalization every time she disobeyed her. She finally had run away, and got into some minor legal difficulties. She was referred by the court to the unit for evaluation, and (as she told it), "the next thing I knew, they were holding me down and frying my brain".

"I used to trust Dr. Joltzer," she offered. "I've been seeing him off and on for two years. He's been trying to get me to agree to these crazy shock treatments, but I told him there was no way. This time, he told me if I didn't sign the consent form, they would take me off to jail . . . Big choice; maybe I'd be better off there . . ." Her voice trailed off into a little-girl whimper. "I feel awful; My head is banging from the inside out, and I feel dizzy. Help me . . ."

I took Ellen's hand with my free arm, and we walked slowly to room 14. It helped her to sit down, but she begged for aspirin. "It was the same the other day. I feel like I want to die after these treatments. Could you please get me some aspirin?"

I assured her I would try, and left. At the nurses' station, aspirin was being dispensed in all directions. "Give me two more, you cheap bastard, It's the least you can do", a man yelled loudly. "It's your damn fault I got this headache."

"Two it is for you, Mr. Green. You know the rules. I can talk to you about it later, if you wish."

"Later, schmater. Later never comes around here. You're all a bunch of damn liars."

"Pay him no mind," the aide whispered to me. "Some of 'em gets real nasty after shock."

I saw to it that Ellen got her two aspirin, and walked around in a daze that entire day. The next day, I returned to orientation in the E.C.T. room. (Maybe Miss Warner was right; I did seem to be a glutton for punishment at times.)

"Nothin' to it," the old aide chuckled. "I been workin' here for years. It ain't what people think it is. Jes' stan' there, and we'll take care of Mr. Green here. He's an old-timer."

"Old-timer, my foot!" he yelled back, sticking out his foot as if to emphasize his point. "You bandits been suckin' my blood for years. This is the last straw, though. I warn you . . ."

He lay down on the cot. They loosened his trousers by undoing the button, and then proceeded, first unbuttoning the top of his shirt, then taking away his glasses, and finally checking his mouth for dentures. "Keep your dirty fingers outta my mouth," his voice bellowed through the halls. "One of these days, I'll bite it off."

The aide laughed. "Your bark's meaner than your bite, Green,"

137

he guffawed, obviously amused at his words. To add insult to injury (literally), he followed with "And besides, you won't be harming a flea when we're done with you."

His massive body was strapped loosely to the cot, and they injected some medication into the vein in his arm. One of the aides held what looked like a black football, explaining that it was an ambu bag, waiting to be pumped full of human breath.

"What's that?" I whispered almost inaudibly, pointing to the injection.

"Curare," he answered curtly. "And a tranquilizer. Stops 'em from breathing for a minute so we can shock 'em."

I had heard of curare. It's muscle paralyzer - I remember we used it to kill frogs in biology class. Their muscles would freeze, and they would suffocate due to lack of breathing. I also recalled hearing once that ancient tribes used to paint their arrows with curare to ensure death.

"Isn't that dangerous?", my voice said softly.

"Naw" was the answer he gave. "We use it all the time."

With that he watched Mr. Green as the doctor came over and turned the dials on the machine attached by wires to the patient's head. Suddenly, Mr. Green's body twitched and jerked (what appeared to be) almost a foot up in the air. "Now ya see why we strap 'em down," he bellowed. "That's a jolt!"

I felt sick. My stomach jumped and contorted with Mr. Green. His feet pointed inward: then, as they used the ambu bag, he emitted a loud wheeze and gasped for air.

"That's all," the aide announced, as I watched the ambu bag pump air into the wracking body. "Told ya there was nothin' to it."

I walked out and gagged in the hall, fighting to keep my breakfast in. Somehow, despite it all, curiosity got the best of me, and I asked all the questions I needed to have answered.

I found out that Dr. Joltzer did not spend much time on the unit, though he was officially in charge of it. Much of his 'patient contact' consisted of communications via the nurses, over the telephone. He operated largely by virtue of 'standing orders', which meant that he had a regular routine prescribed for all his patients. (Hardly an individualized treatment plan). Part of his routine seemed to involve the administration of E.C.T., and his standards for determining who would receive this treatment differed from anything I had ever read or heard.

On several occasions, I had to contact him on the phone about one of his patients. His typical response was "Tell her that I'm not interested in discussing anything further with her until she has received several more treatments."

Dr. Joltzer's rationale seemed to be that the person was not ready to be counselled seriously until some of the severe agitation and depression were relieved. He was extremely impersonal in his interactions, and though I'm anything but shy by nature, I felt very intimidated by him.

His patients, likewise, were afraid of him, and very few spoke out about their treatment - to him. The nurses and aides, on the other hand, were bombarded with the enormous anger and resentments these patients carried. This was a real problem - created by the doctor, but handled by the nurses.

The social worker on the unit, with whom I worked closely, was named Helen. Helen's job was to be in close communication with the patients, to get to know them and observe their progress or lack thereof, and see that they were sent on to an appropriate facility, if need be - or home, if possible.

Since this unit was classified as an acute care center, patients were to receive a disposition within thirty days. Helen had been working on this unit for two years, and as we grew to trust each other, she filled me in on all she had seen.

She informed me that E.C.T. was an *extremely lucrative business,* taking minimal time on the doctors' part for maximum return. It was her feeling that the physicians did not 'waste' their time doing psychotherapy with their patients - that they relied on a 'zap' to do the job quickly.

After E.C.T., the patients did indeed get 'better' if better means less argumentative and less demanding. After several treatments, most of them became docile and glassy-eyed. My attempts to deeply connect were incredibly frustrating. I would work through the initial stages of acquiring mutual respect and trust, and often be able to help them with their anxieties and problems. Then they would go off to their treatment, and come back with that horribly vacant stare.

"Who are you?" one man asked me after I had spent many hours working with him. "Have I ever seen you before?"

What was the use? I soon came to recognize which patients had undergone a long series of shock treatments previously in their psychiatric care. What concerned me the most, however, was an excessive number of young people - often adolescents - who were regularly shocked.

I had been taught that shock was a seldom-applied therapy, most useful for a condition known as 'involutional melancholia', a

140

depression which generally surfaced in middle age. This hardly applied to the many teenagers I witnessed, nor to most of the patients on this unit.

Helen and I decided to keep records of the types of treatments used for patients on this unit. By the end of the summer, our carefully-recorded statistics revealed that 83% of the patients on this unit received E.C.T. I could only believe that she must be right - much of the shock therapy was done for financial reasons.

Third-party payors, like insurance companies or Medicaid-Medicare, paid big money for this treatment, above and beyond the standard charges for inpatient hospitalization and other treatments. Most patients received E.C.T. daily for almost four weeks, and then no more, because third-party coverage paid for it only during the first month of hospitalization.

Needless to say, all of this had me wondering, as I'm highly prone to do anyhow. The therapeutic tool itself was not a villain. Evidently E.C.T. can be an appropriate and helpful technique, under certain conditions.

The third-party payors were not villains. They had devised and were paying for what they must have felt were sensible guidelines for reimbursement of necessary medical procedures.

The doctor was not a villain. He seemed to believe in the heavy application of technological therapies for difficult medical problems, perhaps as taught to him in medical school. In addition, he obviously had the understandable and common desire to make a good living for himself and his family.

The hospital owners/administrators who did the billing and paid the staff were not villains. They apparently needed to run their facility in a well-managed, business-like way (i.e. make a profit), or else go out of business. The nurses and other para-medical staff were not villains. They needed to follow orders or else lose their jobs.

Least of all were the patients or their families villains. They seemed to be innocent pawns in a large and confused chess game. Perhaps, everyone involved in this unfortunate scenario was an innocent pawn to a medical system gone haywire.

If no one is a villain, why is this happening? What's missing from this picture? More than anything, what's missing is a good dose of compassion - and courage. More compassion would shed light on the underlying suffering and dehumanization of all people concerned. More courage would propel some or all of the pawns into the actions necessary for improvement.

If there were a conspiracy - that is, many of us working together to make things better - even a little more compassion and courage could have enormous benefit.

You see, I have observed this very situation over and over in many different settings since those early days. An excess of 'profit motive' and a decrease in 'compassionate caring' makes for bad medicine.

Perhaps you and your loved ones have encountered this theme in other arenas of endeavor. Together, speaking out, we all have a part in changing the experience for the better.

Alone, however, on that psychiatry unit, I was merely able to make a few small waves. Helen was asked to leave the unit shortly after presenting the results of our research, and I left shortly thereafter to resume my studies.

Who knows what 'ripple effects' resulted from our presence

there? Perhaps the statistics managed to turn some heads? Maybe the unit ultimately became even a little more humane as a long-term result of two of us conspiring . . . I certainly hope so, knowing that it can make all the difference.

~   ~   ~   ~   ~

In looking back, I can easily trace the path the led me to become a rabble-rouser. Somehow, I had an uncanny knack for being in the wrong place at the right time, or something like that.

Despite advice to the contrary, I found that my heart and head were permanently connected, and seemed to work together quite nicely. Occasionally, however - without warning - my mouth would slip into gear. My words, my truth as I saw it, would slip out, demanding that the shoe fit who wore it.

Like many separate threads of yarn, each of these encounters became woven into the fabric of my nursing life. Gradually, I was more able to fill in some obvious gaps. The result was a growing tapestry of understanding (with a few loose threads here and there).

One major theme was beginning to emerge above all else. Somehow, the role of the nurse, that mythical angel-healer, was changing in my awareness. Earlier impressions from the days of Miss Warner and nursing homes were being validated.

It was painfully obvious that the contented, dedicated nurse of my dreams and fantasies, and of books, movies and general public awareness were indeed different from the nurses I was meeting. Why such disparity? Which was the real nurse? Most important, had the nurses made conscious choices as to how they would work with patients, or were they unconscious victims of a steamrolling medical system - a runaway monster which flattened out their dreams and

143

infuriated their soul?

I had to find out . . .

Postscript

In the years since I acquired my MS in Psychiatric Nursing, I have held several positions in Psychiatry, including being involved in the creation of a specialized day treatment program for chronic schizophrenic retarded young adults. Though I loved this position, I became overly involved, (a common occupational hazard) and eventually left to try to balance my life out more by becoming Impatient Unit Coordinator of a psychiatric unit in a rural hospital.

Several years later I moved out to California, where again I worked in a day treatment facility, then later hemodialysis. I left institutional nursing in 1976. My healing journey led me to volunteer time at a holistic health center, where I learned about natural healing modalities, and met my life partner (there are definite advantages to following one's heart and instincts).

We moved to Hawaii in 1978 to write our first book together, and we now have three beautiful children and maintain a collaborative holistic practice. Our work is exciting, rewarding and joyful. I encourage every person to follow the 'path with a heart', for therein lies your treasure.

PART III

WHAT IS THE SOLUTION?

PATHWAYS TO RECOVERY

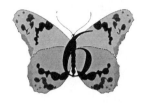

HOLISTIC HEALTH
NURSING'S ORIGINAL VISION RE-EMERGES

I recently read the beautiful textbook, *Holistic Nursing*.[25] Textbooks rarely provide me with emotional experiences, but much of this one did.

In this book, Dr. Lynn Keegan[26] has outlined the history of healing with an unusual slant:

> ". . . from the very earliest times, healers have used their creative force to explore and utilize everything that their time and culture afforded them to augment the still-mysterious healing process . . ."[27]

> "People living in primitive cultures were closely tied into natural law . . . believed that all natural objects . . . were alive and possessed a spirit or soul . . . believed

illness might be due to spiritual woes . . ."[28]

"Many scholars date the beginning of the Scientific Revolution to the work of the 17th-century philosopher Rene Descartes . . . Spirit, in the form of God, hovers on the outside of the universe, but plays no direct part in it . . . it was this duality of thinking, the heart of the Cartesian paradigm, that broke the body-mind-spirit connection."[29]

"By the 19th-century the Cartesian approach was well-integrated into the healing arts. Both physicians and nurses followed scientific curricula and worked diligently to serve the sick using their best atomistic approaches . . ."[30]

"It was, however, during the second half of the 19th-century when . . . ultimate dissolution of the feminine influence on medicine occurred. As the scientific content of nursing curricula increased, the feminine qualities of nurturance, intuition, and empathy decreased . . ."[31]

". . . In the late 19th- and first half of the 20th-centuries, the increasing division between the healers (doctors and nurses) and increasing specialization . . . pushed the concept of whole body healing farther and farther into the recess of the past."[32]

"With the exception of the isolated work of a few healers, by the 1960's the pendulum had swung the limit away from holistic health care. Illness was perceived as a strictly pathophysiologic event . . ."[33]

150

Dr. Keegan next follows the reawakening of the holistic movement, starting with the psychosomatic medicine work of Flanders Dunbar,[34] a psychiatrist at Columbia Presbyterian Medical Center. Later, Hans Seyle[35] explored the general adaptation syndrome and devised a theory of stress. In the 1960's, researchers Holmes and Rahe[36] found a correlation between lifestyle events, and onset of illness.

One of the major advances in the concept of 'wellness' occurred in the early 1960's, when Halbert L. Dunn MD,[37] described the importance of inspiring each person to reach his or her maximum aliveness in her own environment. Then, in 1974, the Canadian Ministry of Health and Welfare issued "A New Perspective on the Health of Canadians",[38] which supported the important connection between environment and health. Two years later, the U.S. government released a vital report[39] (Senate Select Committee on Nutrition and Human Needs), attempting to improve the dangerous eating habits of Americans.

The late 1970's witnessed an explosion of information and interest in the holisitic model, with seed centers springing up to support conscious consumerism in relation to nutrition, stress reduction, physical awareness, and self-responsibility. Literature and research began to emerge, influencing the awareness of the American public.

In 1980, Marilyn Ferguson's *Aquarian Conspiracy*[40] described a transformation taking place, a new paradigm that allowed for an expanded view of human inter-relatedness and potential in all fields of endeavor. She described major differences between the old and new paradigms of medicine:

Old Paradigm of Medicine	New Paradigm of Medicine
Treatment of symptoms specialized	Search for patterns and causes, plus symptoms, Integrated; concerned with the whole patient
Emphasis on efficiency	Emphasis on human values
Professional should be emotionally neutral	Professional's 'caring' is a component of healing
Pain and disease are wholly negative	Pain and disease are information about conflict, disharmony
Primary intervention with drugs, surgery	Minimal intervention 'appropriate technology', complemented with full armamentarium of non-invasive techniques (psy-chotherapies, diet, and exercise)
Body seen as machine in good or bad repair	Body seen as dynamic system, context, field of energy within other fields
Disease or disability seen as thing	Disease or disability seen as process

Old Paradigm of Medicine	New Paradigm of Medicine
Emphasis on eliminating symptoms	Emphasis on maximum wellness
Patient is dependent	Patient is (should be) autonomous
Professional is authority	Professional is therapeutic partner
Body and Mind are separate; psychosomatic illness is mental illness - may be referred to psychiatrist	Body-mind perspective; psychosomatic illness is province of all health-care professionals
Mind is secondary factor in organic illness	Mind is primary or coequal factor in all illness
Placebo effect shows power of suggestion	Placebo effect shows mind's role in disease and healing
Primary reliance on quantitative information (charts, test, dates)	Primary reliance on qualitative information, including patient's subjective reports and professionals' intuition; quantitative data an adjunct
'Prevention' largely environmental: vitamins, rest, exercise, immunization, not smoking	'Prevention' synonymous with wholeness, work [41]

Also in 1980, the American Holistic Nurses Association was created with the intent to educate nurses and the public about whole-person healing. Through this growing organization, thousands of nurses have created a powerful and loving community, dedicated to healing themselves and the planet. Together, nurses are bringing alive the concepts of holism, and finding the support and creativity which enables them to move in powerful new directions in their work. Together, we are weaving a strong foundation for a new vision of nursing.

In Canada, the Canadian Holistic Nurses Association continues to expand, and other groups are forming in Australia and New Zealand. There are numerous other organizations dedicated to holistic principles, including the American Holistic Medical Association[42] and Nurse-Healers Professional Associates,[43] to name only a few.

Just what are the problems we seek to ameliorate by returning to a more holistic framework? We can now explore the numerous challenges before us as nurses approaching the 21st-century.

The New Paradigm

We live in a time of profound change and rapid transition. When we consider the magnitude of the challenges upon us, we can wonder where to begin. From the holistic framework, we need to examine physical, mental, emotional and spiritual levels.

Our physical environment suffers severe ecological deterioration from both neglect and abuse. There is distressing pollution of our water and air. In addition, we find an alarming variety of poten-

154

tially harmful chemicals in our food.

Our psychological environment shows equally serious symptoms. The number of divorces exceeds the number of marriages in some areas. Widespread job dissatisfaction, unemployment, frighteningly high drug use and rampant crime express a growing sense of restlessness and alienation.

On the spiritual level, people appear to have less sense of connection to a power greater than themselves. With the lessening influence of traditional religion, there seems to be little else to fill the void for most people. The result for many is a gnawing sense of confusion and lack.

It certainly feels as if our survival as a species is being threatened. On the brighter side, however, these enormous challenges on the physical, mental, and emotional levels are inspiring individuals to learn specific tools for adapting to change.

It is in response to this need for maintaining personal sanity and continuing survival that a new, shared consciousness (or conscience) is beginning to emerge. In fact, health is only one expression of this new consciousness. Across the country and in various parts of the world, we see accelerated research in such areas as ecology, conservation, human potential, psychology, parapsychological phenomena, and mystical religion. Yet as we open our eyes to our future potentials, we are also forced to take a hard look at our current American health care system, and consider the medicine of other cultures.

For instance, the medical and spiritual traditions of China and India for thousands of years have viewed the person as a unified energy system, existing in meaningful, interdependent relationship with the world environment.

Holistic approaches to health still exist today in most of the East and in various 'primitive' societies. Holism can refer to the blend of old and new, East and West, and incorporates a mind-body-spirit perspective.

The American Indian culture offers a good example. For the Native American, the term 'medicine' meant even more than overall health care. Various psychological and cosmological events, such as an eclipse, were viewed as either good or bad medicine, depending on their entire context. Medicine was the flow of the physical and spiritual universe rather than merely an ingredient to temporarily alter a body function.

Such all-encompassing perspectives, however, have lacked a precise knowledge of specific processes, such as blood circulation, hormone control, or psychological defense mechanisms. Thus, the 'forest' had been seen clearly, while knowledge of the 'trees' remained a mystery.

On the other hand, Western society has taken until recently a mechanistic, part-by-part approach. The dualistic concept of 'mind' versus 'body', for example, is a Western invention. Researchers schooled in this form of thought have become specialists in the most minute facets of human functioning. For instance, it is well known that Western physicians often focus on only one part of the body, or on one type of illness, and consider the larger picture as beyond their domain. Ivan Illich, a controversial sociologist, suggested some years ago in his book *Medical Nemesis*[44] that the medical industry may cause a great deal of the suffering that it cures. By this he meant much more than simply that doctors can make mistakes and that 'wonder drugs' can have serious side effects. All this is true, and in addition, we are being subliminally trained to ignore our innate

156

capacity to heal ourselves.

We have given up the healthy autonomy of self-reliance and traded it for a less healthy overdependence on healers and external chemicals. We consume enormous amounts of legally sanctioned chemicals ranging from stomach and headache relievers to mood elevators and energy stimulants. It is estimated that seventy million Americans (one-third of the population) regularly rely on medications of some sort.

We notoriously spend vast sums of money treating all kinds of preventable disease. To make matters worse, hospital and physician costs are skyrocketing. Moreover, while more conscientious doctors and nurses are needed, many are discouraged from working due to outrageous malpractice insurance premiums.

Yet in the midst of the need to reevaluate and restructure our questionable health systems, politicians are urging the extension of availability rather than also asking for better quality. In fact, only a tiny fraction of our entire health budget is spent on prevention.

In addition to these political realities, and perhaps underlying them, is another fundamental problem in our thinking about health - health and health care are not the same. Researchers have discovered that health is only minimally affected by health care. Other factors, both personal and environmental, have a far greater impact on one's overall well-being than most health practitioners have been willing to acknowledge.

Any such extreme polarity creates a tension that calls for synthesis. We are experiencing this today in the field of health care. Recent developments point toward an emerging synthesis that combines the Eastern emphasis on understanding the whole with the

Western emphasis on understanding the part. This emerging new approach emphasizes compassion and humanism as a key way to bring greater balance between physical, mental, and spiritual realms.

For nurses to empower consumers with this expanded view, we must first each embark on this healing journey, putting ourselves in charge of our own well-being. As we demonstrate that we can indeed be in charge of our own medical fate, we become believable as role models.

Inner Wisdom: Our Personal Healing Guidance

We each possess a health-oriented inner wisdom that can and will guide us if we let it. It is part of our tissues and microbiochemistry, including the intricate wiring of our brain. It expresses our long evolutionary adaptation and our deep spiritual nature.

This unconscious knowledge has greater self-healing ability than the conscious mind of everyday life. It cannot be lied to or tricked. It always has our best interest at heart. It is the source of those messages called *intuition.*

Consider the example: "Although he spoke convincingly, I had a funny feeling about that broker from the beginning. I'm glad I didn't invest with him because it turned out that he was a swindler."

Here is a similar experience: "Right as I took that medicine, I had the notion that something was wrong. It wasn't a pain or an upset stomach. It was just a vague concern. Instead of taking more, I called the doctor, and sure enough, the prescription was not filled correctly. If I had taken it all, I might have died."

Still another example was once expressed by a patient. "When I first got married, everyone wanted me to go into my father-in-law's business, and I do mean everyone. Logically, it was the smartest thing to do, and he was a generous, non-interfering man. Even though I didn't have any idea how to go about it, I just felt like sticking to my plans for a career in music. Now I thank my lucky stars I did it my way."

Whether we realize it or not, the inner wisdom operates all the time. The world's greatest scientists and educators have talked about it through the ages. Some have called it *the ghost within the machine.* This is in reference to that invisible creativity that seems to pervade our biological mechanisms. Others refer to it as *the vital force*, the underlying drive that organizes and balances one's life processes.

Scientists and physicians who could not believe in an unseen force invented their own name. They called it homeostasis. This medical term, which means 'to stay the same', describes the body's self-maintenance of an inner equilibrium. Temperature, breathing, digestion, and circulation, all seem to run on 'automatic pilot'.

Nobel Prize winner Albert Saint-George went even further when he wrote about *the drive in living matter to perfect itself.* In his view, all living cells have an innate interest in better and better functioning. Just as a species tends to perfect itself over many generations, the individual develops greater perfection during his or her own lifetime.

A health-related name given to this internal wisdom is the *three-million-year-old healer.* This concept suggests that each of us is, in effect, a very wise and very old healer, having bodily knowledge about fighting illness that goes back to the dawn of human life

159

on this planet. Our immune system prevents and fights infections, and cut fingers and broken bones seem to know how to heal themselves. Both a cold and a heart attack are best treated by simply going to bed and resting completely. Most depressions recover on their own in four to six months regardless of medical treatment.

Each of the above major concepts - the ghost within the machine, the vital force, homeostasis, the drive in the living matter to perfect itself, and *the three million year old healer* - expresses in a unique fashion the same reality: the wisdom necessary for true health lies within. We may do well to put ourselves in our own hands. As nurses, if we can learn to rely more and more on our own internal wisdom, we will not only come to understand and appreciate our body's innate wisdom, but we can truly inspire our patients with the examples we set.

An Example 'Close to Home'

To bring this concept alive, I would like to share the story of my three most profound life experiences, my births. Not only do they reflect a belief in a deep internal wisdom, but they also demonstrate how we can empower ourselves in such a way as to provide a model for others.

Prior to having children, my mate Richard and I were living in Hawaii, where we wrote a book together. Several months after we conceived, I had a dream and awoke that morning with a start. In the dream, there was a woman with dark eyes and a graying bun, looking right into my eyes. "Phoenix - you go to Phoenix". I jumped from the bed.

"Phoenix. What do you *mean* Phoenix? Phoenix, Arizona? I

160

don't want to go to Phoenix, Arizona. Why in the world would I leave one of the most beautiful islands imaginable to land in a built-up desert?" Rich asked what I was mumbling about. "There was a lady in the dream telling me to go to Phoenix." He thought about it.

"Well," he said pensively, "the only thing I know about Phoenix is that it's the home of a well-known holistic medical clinic. There's a very special woman doctor there who has developed a 'baby buggy' program, with a mobile home-birthing unit. Maybe our baby wants to be born there."

I'll spare you all the miraculous details. Suffice it to say, we ended up in Phoenix in time for the birth. The great surprise, for me, was to meet this special woman doctor - she was the spitting image of the woman in my dream! She cared for me during the duration of my pregnancy, along with a nurse-midwife. When my contractions began to come on strong, they both joined Richard and me with several other dear friends. Throughout the pregnancy, they had inspired me to stay in close contact with the soul of the being who had chosen to come through me. (They very much believed in past lives). Though initially it seemed strange, after I learned more about dream interpretation through a special program they offered, I must say that it certainly seemed to all make sense. I truly enjoyed the experience of learning about birth from these beautiful teachers.

In contrast, I could recall my own obstetrical training experiences at an Armed Forces center in Virginia. There, the pregnant women were treated like cattle. They lined up in front of a scale, recorded their weight, sat in stuffy, crowded waited rooms, and were frequently scolded by noxious overweight and overworked doctors who told them they gained too much - or not enough - weight. It was ludicrous, really, now that I recall the scene. There was one doctor there who was prone to having regular tantrums in the delivery room. While women were struggling to deliver their babies, he would get upset if the nurse didn't hand him the equipment fast enough and would throw the speculum against the wall and yell obscenities.

Gladys and Doris taught me that every birth is perfect for each mother and baby. Needless to say, my situation was perfect for me. During my birth, while I was gently laboring in the peace and serenity of my own home, there was a knock at the door. In walked our neighbor, an obstetrics resident. He thought I was joking when I said I was in labor, though he was curious about that big pink and blue van parked out front.

Dr. Gladys took him aside, and started whispering the secrets of the ages into his ear while the nurse attended to me. I chanted, I meditated, we sang softly, candles were lit as I took an inward journey to find my inner guidance and prepare for the miraculous event at hand. When I went deep within my being, I made a strong contact with my baby, and felt very holy. The presence and constant support of these loving, skilled caregivers eased any fears from my mind. It was so very different from the masculine medical model, and I knew innately that this was how birth was intended to be, by women, with women, with a deep inner trust in the beauty of our bodies and the process.

Through their compassion, I was continually and gently reminded to follow in the footsteps of women since time began. When it was time to push, I gave one push and out popped my brave and beautiful daughter, Shauna. She is exactly who I knew she was, and when my sister's plane finally landed in Phoenix, and she breathlessly came rushing in hopes of attending the birth, I walked to the front door with Shauna in my arms and an enormous grin on my face. It was only a few minutes after delivery. My birth was indeed perfect for us.

A year after this birth, we were living in the mountains of Northern California when I got an insatiable urge to have another child. Rich weakly protested at first, eventually succumbing to the pressure to try again. Within weeks, I felt very pregnant, though Rich seemed certain that I was dreaming. He took a urine sample to his office and tested it, then announced that it was negative. We repeated this several times, each with the same results.

Deep in my heart, in my heart of hearts where all answers to our lives lie, I *knew* beyond any doubt that I was pregnant. They call this 'women's intuition', yet I believe we all possess this ability, were we to learn to trust and develop it more.

Finally, we decided to load up our camper and head to the ocean for a few healing days. At a most spectacular and wild Northern California beach, with wild elk all around, I sat at the ocean's edge and prayed for guidance. I felt very pregnant, and wondered what was going on. I asked for a sign to show me the truth, and within a minute I found myself doubled over on the beach, heaving the contents of my stomach. Then I was sure. I ran up the steps to the camper, screaming "I am, I am. I knew I was."

Richard stuck his head out of the camper to see what the commotion was all about. When I told him, he look puzzled. "Then why are your urine tests coming up negative?" he asked. I did not have an answer to this, but challenged him to drive to the nearest community clinic with me to check it out. We drove to a nearby town, where my pregnancy test was positive!

163

Then my answer was shown to me. Rich's face fell, and he looked very worried. When I asked him what was the matter, he told me that, on deeper reflection, he didn't feel ready for another baby. He felt sure the timing was wrong for our family, and therefore had been hoping against hope that I wasn't pregnant.

I was devastated. We usually saw eye to eye on things, and this was a big one for me. I was angry and felt betrayed at this late confession. I felt frightened about how we would resolve it. It was a test for our marriage.

After a few days of soul-searching, I saw that he was very definite about his feelings. After moving through my fear, and some anger, I decided to seek the wisdom of my body for a solution. I have learned more and more that the body can be an ally when considered such.

In my meditation, I was told that I could communicate with the soul of the baby, and elicit it's support. I then communed with the forming baby inside, suggesting that it consider leaving now and coming back in another six or eight months, when Shauna was older and felt more secure.

It was not a total surprise when, upon returning home from our trip, I noticed the gushing blood that signified the end of the pregnancy. Though I was sad, and Rich and I had to work through the feelings, I knew that it couldn't be right ultimately unless we both agreed on it.

Eight months later, also after meditating and praying to be granted the privilege of bringing in another soul, I became pregnant - again on the very first try, much to my husband's chagrin. He had certainly hoped to take more time trying!

164

This time, we were living in Santa Barbara, as my Gypsy nature dictated. I made arrangements for emergency medical care, then chose as my primary attendants two lay midwives who were nurses. They were so gentle and loving to me and our family unity, and I felt as comfortable and relaxed as possible with a bustling two-year old as well.

My midwives this time were Wendy and Merrily. Merrily, my dear friend, lived in Hawaii and planned to do the delivery. Wendy, on the other hand, lived in Santa Barbara, and was the one I met with at regular intervals to share my feelings and progress. She was such a loving and compassionate person, and encouraged me to bring Rich and Shauna to our appointments.

She did a very thorough physical examination, checking my urine, blood, blood pressure, listening to the baby's heartbeat, and checking the developmental progress of the fetus. These are the very things obstetricians do routinely. However, what I loved about working with a nurse and midwife was the care I received above and beyond the routine physical care. It was almost as if, after we did the necessary preliminaries, we could move on to the really important issues.

"How are you three doing together?" Wendy would begin. From there we'd move on to my attitude, how I could improve it when necessary, and how my friends could support me. Together we would create positive affirmations that I wrote down and repeated during the coming days, to counterbalance any fears or negative thinking (some examples were "I'm loveable," when I felt irritable, and "our baby is a divine expression of our love" whenever fear showed its unwelcome face).

Believe me, the medical schools could use some courses in

compassion taught by midwives or nurses such as this! I felt so very loved and cared for, I almost hated to see the pregnancy end.

One week prior to my due date, I was enjoying a magnificent ride down the California coast with my dear friend Merrily, who had finally arrived from Hawaii. She suggested we stop for a few minutes. I pulled over and got out of the car, bent over to smell some flowers, and felt a remotely familiar 'pop' in my belly. As I tried to remember when I had felt the funny feeling before, I felt something else - a gush of warm liquid shooting down my legs. Since my water hadn't broken during the first birth until I was near the end of labor, I didn't know whether this was really it or not, though I had my suspicions. Then again, maybe the pressure from this watermelon-sized baby was forcing me to lose control over my bladder.

"Merrily," I ventured in a shaky voice. "I think my water may have broken." Her answer surprised me. "Well, does it taste salty?" I wondered what had gotten into her.

"Merrily, I didn't taste it!" I answered shrilly.

"Well go ahead and try it. If it's salty, it's amniotic fluid."

Can you imagine a doctor saying anything like that? Physicians used to be more like that until this runaway technology distanced them. Nowadays they just are not trained to be attuned on those subtle levels to the natural innate healing wisdom of the body. Hopefully, as more women enter medicine, it will become more and more reverent towards women.

In Hawaii, I had attended a number of home births with Merrily, and I knew that she was the one I wanted to have care for me if at all possible. When she offered to come to the mainland and deliver my second baby, I was delighted. Though she was not a certified nurse-midwife, she had read everything she could to learn about natural ways to have babies. She had worked in obstetrics in hospitals, had studied birth practices in various cultures, and had learned from homeopaths and naturopaths. Her gentle techniques left me no doubt as to their safety, and I trusted her totally.

The birth, likewise, was wonderful. It was very quick this time; I prayed and meditated briefly. Then the contractions seemed to come hot and heavy. Suddenly, I yelled, "I have to push." Before they could get me into the bedroom to check me, there was a head coming out. A girl's body soon followed. "Oh, Georjana, I love you!"

I had done my best to prepare Shauna for all the changes, and had informed her that soon she would have a playmate. That was all interesting to her until the advent of this tiny, red, squalling being. She then looked at me as if I was crazy. "Mom, I can't play with her! She's not even a child." Needless to say, it took all Merrily's and my nursing skills to keep her from playing ball (with her new sister as the ball) in the days to come.

They did, however, learn to love each other, and it was four years later when we decided to try again. This was a difficult decision. In order to make it properly, we agreed to take a nine-month preconception period, one in which I would monitor my body to ascertain exactly when I was ovulating, for we decided to try the natural methods to ensure a male. I felt curious about boys, and knew I could benefit from the experience of raising one.

I learned from the book *How to Choose the Sex of Your Baby*,[45] how to increase our chances for a male, and it took a fair amount of organization. (Not the most romantic process in the world, but after having the first two 'romantically', we felt fine about some plan-

167

ning). After nine months, Rich and I took a weekend at our favorite hot springs resort, and it was there that we conceived our third child. Within eight days after the first attempt, I was hugging the bowl . . .

There was a scary part near the beginning, as our back-up doctor suggested that since I was thirty-seven this time, I should definitely consider having an amniocentesis. Most people consider this a fairly benign procedure, though it carries a risk of miscarriage. I have learned to leave well enough alone whenever possible, and to trust the natural process. I called Merrily to ask for some good nursely advice.

"Ask for guidance," came the voice over the wire all the way from Hawaii. "Before you go to sleep, ask whether you need to have an amniocentesis, then write down what your dreams tell you."

I did this, and had one of the most profound and remarkable dreams of my life. In the dream, Rich and I were attending a conference. I felt a warm gush, and noticed a slight amount of blood coming down my legs. I strongly called Rich into the room, and he was (as often) absorbed in deep conversation. By the time I was able to pull him away from his conversation, I had to lay down quickly, and the baby's head slipped out of the womb, and came through the birth canal and out to see us.

It came out up to the umbilicus, then stopped. First, it stared lovingly right into Rich's eyes, and then turned its head ever so slowly and looked me in the eye. Never had I seen a more perfect and serene face. With a smile and a hint of mischief in its eyes, it slowly twisted and worked its way back up into the womb.

I was left breathless with the distinct memory of that calm, healthy, loving being. When I gathered my thoughts, I laughed. That

168

little stinker - wouldn't even let me see what sex it was! I just knew (once again, that inner voice) that indeed he was the perfect little boy I had prayed for, and I also realized that by asking for the dream, I had managed to avert a costly medical procedure that does carry its risks. I had received a 'dream-amnio', and felt a deep inner sense of calm about delivering a healthy baby.

When the due date came closer, and Merrily once again arrived from Hawaii for the final weeks, I felt totally relaxed and prepared. At her advice, I had resumed my exercise program toward the end. (I had curtailed it for three weeks because I was dilated early, and we all agreed it was best for the baby to stay in a few weeks more).

It was almost Richard's birthday, and I had told him that I thought a birth on his birthday would be a wonderful present. Ever since we had conceived, I felt that was a distinct possibility. I was unprepared for Rich's response. "I'm not sure I'd like that," he said. "I think we should each have our own birthdays." I also felt at that moment that the baby had changed his plan.

I don't know whether it was the blissful jog down Mt. Tamalpais, or the bumpy bicycle ride the next day, but somewhere around that time, Gabriel got the message that it was O.K. to come out. It had been a strange day around our household.

That night, before bed, Shauna, then seven, burst out crying at bedtime, her body wracked with uncontrollable sobbing. "What is it, Shauna?" Rich and I had both tried to figure it out. "I don't know," she had answered. "I just feel like I'm losing something; besides, I never had a brother before." Rich and I looked at each other in puzzlement. (In looking back, I can see that it was her inner wisdom helping to prepare her for the change.)

Also, Rich and I had been quarreling about something that evening, and went to bed unresolved. I remember leaning over and kissing him on the ear and telling him that it was time to let it all go. "Why" he asked. "Because," I had said, "What baby would want to be born with its parents mad at each other?" He hugged me, then as he was drifting off to sleep, I got up, brought something in from the bathroom, and rustled about, fixing the bedcovers.

"What are you doing?" he asked. "I'm putting one of these waterproof pads under me," I said, "just in case the baby should decide to come during the night. I'm hoping it'll happen like last time - and my water will break first. I liked that." I drifted off to sleep in his arms, only to wake up thirty minutes later in a big puddle. "Get up, Rich. It worked. Baby's coming."

We woke Merrily up, and she called our special friends as planned. One by one they came, and I heard them, but was too busy concentrating as I labored in my big clawfoot bathtub. That was the ultimate comfort (if there's any such thing in labor). The warm water seemed to relax and stretch the perineum, and also seemed to absorb most of my contractions. In less than an hour, I felt that familiar need to push. I ran for the bed, and jumped on with my knees together in fetal position. My midwives touched me gently as I yelled "It's coming. What should I do?"

Softly, one of them reminded me. "It's your baby, Karilee. Open your legs. Your baby wants to be born."

Oh, is that what it was? I had almost forgotten. I opened my knees, and down slipped a baby, right into the loving midwife's hands. I knew what it looked like without looking.

"Well, Rich what is it?" I asked dreamily from my pillow.

170

"It's a - boy. Karilee, it's a boy." His face was radiant, and so was everyone else's as they joined us in silent welcome. Gabriel nursed gently, then his older sister cut his cord. His father took him into a fresh warm bath, while the midwives helped me to get cleaned up. There was loving celebration once again in our busy household, as breakfast was cooked and family reunited.

It was the ultimate natural high. I loved being able to receive my children in the dimly-lit comfort of my own home. I loved having the power to orchestrate my birth exactly as I dreamed it could be. I loved knowing that I had all the wisdom needed within me to go through these precious life passages. Most of all, *I loved receiving such loving care from these fine nurses. It made all the difference in my life.*

I had been with a number of women giving birth in hospitals, and invariably things seem to go haywire in that setting. Often, the doctor would rush in, cup of coffee in hand, and start restlessly urging that the baby come out soon. I have seen them look impatiently at their watches, sip coffee, and then order Pitocin. It is almost as if the process has nothing to do with the woman, or her baby, but instead has everything to do with the doctor, and his schedule.

After having the privilege of birthing my three beautiful children at home, with friends supporting us and my husband breathing with me and looking into my eyes. I can't tell you of the pain in my heart when, as a therapist, I listen to many woman cry over their birth experiences. I can assure you their sadness is deep and lengthy. Many carry a constant ache in their heart. One example is Julie.

Julie had been planning a home birth for her second child. Towards the end, she was in very good spirits, even though the baby was late. After about a week, her doctor said he wanted to electri-

171

cally monitor the baby to be sure everything was all right. Though she was shaky about doing this, she eventually succumbed to the pressure.

Her experience was anything but pleasant. The doctor said that the test was slightly irregular, and that he didn't know what it meant. By now, of course, she was very worried and anxious. She began to show a rapid heartbeat, and the doctor then told her that her increased pulse rate could adversely affect the baby. Many of you can guess the end of this story. They cut the baby out by Caesarian section.

Though Julie was in love with her new daughter, she had difficulty bonding with her. In counseling sessions, the wellspring of feelings ran on and on. She was angry at the doctor for frightening her unnecessarily. She was angry at the baby for being born Caesarian section. (Yes, it's irrational, and it happens. Emotions are not rational!)

Most of all, she was angry at herself for succumbing to the pressures. She felt like less of a woman for not being able to give birth vaginally, and hated her body with its enormous surgical scar. To her, it represented a lifetime reminder of her fallen dreams.

I have talked to many women who feel this way after a C-section birth. Thirty years ago the rates for Caesarians was negligible, and recently they've accounted for almost 40% of births in some hospitals. I feel certain that doctors have no idea of the tremendous disservice they are doing when they indiscriminately perform Caesarians. Many seem to sincerely believe that C-sections are somehow more medically indicated these days.

It is obviously a more lucrative endeavor for the physician and hospital, since a lot of money can be gained for minimal time expenditure. There is no long wait. It's neat; it's 'safe'; and somehow we've become convinced that it's normal!

Have we lost our minds? When specific populations can receive proper prenatal care and support, and deliver babies with no medication or intervention more than 95% of the time, how could we allow the medical system to convince us that the best thing to do is to cut one of every four babies out?

In her scathing new book *Backlash: The Undeclared War Against American Women,* author Susan Faludi discusses the issue of male control in birthing.

> "Doctors who had first defined the fetus as an independent patient with a right to treatment, now began to define the pregnant woman as an ancillary party with no right to refuse treatment. First, the doctors had issued a list of prohibitions, telling pregnant women what they couldn't do with their own bodies. Then the doctors went on the offensive, telling pregnant women that physicians would now be free to operate on their bodies - with or without their consent. In a 1986 national survey of directors of maternal-fetal medicine fellowship programs, nearly half the doctors said they supported court orders that forced pregnant women to submit to obstetrical procedures - and favored involuntary detention of pregnant women whose failure to submit, they believe, might pose a risk to the fetus. Less than a quarter consistently supported a competent pregnant woman's right to refuse her doctor's orders . . ."[46]

Another Personal Story

Recently, women have begun to question this, and many who were previously delivered by Caesarian have opted to try for vaginal delivery, often with little support from their obstetricians. I worked with one such woman when I lived in rural northern California years ago.

Angela asked me to provide some birth support for her second birth experience. She had a six - year old son, and was seven months pregnant when I began to do emotional release counseling with her. She had some very specific fears related to the experiences she had during her first delivery, which had turned out to be Caesarian. She desperately sought to heal herself of this previous experience by delivering vaginally (at home if possible) for her second birth.

As the due date arrived, there was an exciting air of anticipation in her household. She was fully prepared to deliver vaginally with the local midwives, as long as all signs indicated that the baby was not in distress. Several weeks passed, and Angela did not go into labor. She was still small, and thought perhaps there was a miscalculation of her due date. She had always taken great care of her body, with natural foods and plenty of exercise and positive thinking. A simple and spiritual woman, she was most comfortable allowing nature to take its course.

Her doctor, on the other hand, became very upset and nervous, even though the vital signs for both mother and baby were totally normal. He applied an external monitor, and though the results seemed within normal limits, he began to pressure Angela to enter the hospital and be induced.

Three weeks after the due date, Angela called me in tears. She

174

said her doctor was insisting that she check herself into the hospital the next day to be internally monitored. She felt instinctively that everything was all right, and wanted to wait for her body to initiate the birth process. She asked if I would come over and do a session with her.

I went over at dinner time, telling my family I'd be back shortly. When I arrived, Angela was undeniably upset. I had her lay on her bed, and put her hands on her bulging belly. I asked her to close her eyes, take some slow deep breaths, and concentrate on contacting her inner wisdom and the baby's spirit. After several minutes, she seemed peaceful and relaxed.

I then guided her through a brief visualization process, to enable her to see her baby. After this, I asked her if there was anything she needed to say to the baby. She began to sob heavily, and told her baby that she was very sorry that she had so much fear; that her first birth had been so traumatic that she was afraid to go through another birth experience; that she knew she could deliver naturally and wanted that more than anything in the world. As she spoke these words, her water broke, and before we knew it, Angela was having strong contractions. I quickly called her midwives, and my family, and told them I wouldn't be home that night - that a baby was about to be born. It was a wonderful and very peaceful home birth.

Angela's husband and son supported the midwives, and I gently massaged her, whispering positive affirmations to her softly. She laughed, she cried, and she told the baby she was no longer afraid and that it could come out. Within a few hours, a beautiful baby girl slid out of her body.

Needless to say, it was a very surprised doctor who greeted Angela and her new baby girl the next morning when she showed up

175

for her appointment. He was actually very curious about how this had all occurred, and Angela spent a long time gently informing him of the previous day's events. She felt powerful and healed for giving herself the opportunity to make her own dreams come true. In addition, she felt that in sharing the experience with her doctor, she might be helping other women under his care, women who might then have more chance of doing their births their own way.

Becoming One's Own Master

Now that we have a general impression, and some very personal examples, of how the inner wisdom can guide us towards our own health, we can explore more fully how it operates. We can begin to grasp a more expanded concept of 'health' to incorporate the less tangible, yet very influential, realms of emotions and spirituality. We can see that the American medical system has missed a most essential ingredient in caring for the person only on the body level, neglecting the opportunities to inspire a complete healing.

If all healing is basically self-healing, then doctors and drugs merely act as catalysts, except in the most extreme situations. Even in those extreme instances, we often find that patients do well or do poorly because of their will to live. How often have you heard that the "operation was a success, but the patient died", usually referring to a failure to inspire the inner drive of the person to keep the machine going.

Sometimes, on the other hand, the situation is reversed, and the doctor says: "The odds were against her ever walking again, but by amazing strength of will she overcame the obstacles." Such occurrences are common and suggest a simple yet often ignored principle.

176

Whether a person gets better or worse is almost entirely up to that person. Healing ultimately has much more to do with one's attitude than with any outside agent or therapist.

This facet of the inner wisdom is what holistic practitioners have referred to as the will to be well. It is simply the old will to live, operating on a milder day-to-day basis. Consciously developing *the will to be well* is the first step in staying healthy or in healing oneself. It involves *choosing* optimistic, relaxing thoughts over pessimistic, tension-provoking ones. At each and every moment, we have this choice. The more we allow and encourage the positive thoughts, the more we develop the will to be well. In addition to the physical dimension of cuts and bruises, the inner wisdom works on the psychological dimension and can be consulted in a similar way.

Unexpected Changes

Patients do immeasurably better when they seek out and relate to the inner wisdom rather than merely depend on external sources. Take, for example, the following discussion at a group meeting where a client named Claudia explained the debilitating effect of overdependence on outside guidance.

"Before I began to trust my own inner wisdom, my health was a mess. I was totally dependent on doctors for everything. I depended on them to tell me if I was sick or well and what I should do about it. I had no confidence in my own healing capabilities. Also, I felt like the unlucky victim of whatever illness came along rather than a consenting accomplice. I had this helpless feeling about myself. Often one illness would lead to another. The antibiotics for my strep throats always gave me a yeast infection. The yeast medicine would

177

give me a skin allergy. Not being able to have intercourse depressed me."

Another example is offered by a twenty-two year old art student who I counseled in my office. Jane had talent in her chosen field, but was always worried about competition and productivity. Her latest medical problem was severe gas, stomach pain, and constipation. Visits to conventional doctors and over-the-counter remedies were only of minimal help. Her tests were all normal; no disease was detectable. Yet her stomach would often swell with painful gas, and she would generally have to strain to move her bowels. Laxatives and stool softeners began to clutter her bathroom cabinet. Next, she developed hemorrhoids.

Someone had suggested that it was her nerves and that she should take hot baths twice a day to relax. She did this and found that her constipation and tension grew worse, as she began to scratch nervously and developed patches of itchy red skin. Jane also felt bewildered by her uncontrollable situation. She was already some-what depressed about her predicament when she came to see me.

Such a situation is common when one has become insensitive to feedback from within. In both of the above cases, a sense of helplessness had developed. Attention to one's inner world can often reinstate the lost feeling of self-control. One then might be able to diagnose and even cure one's own health problems.

Here is how Jane did it. She attended a class on self-healing and learned a technique for consulting her inner wisdom. The activity was a simple meditative process that had profound effects for her. She would merely imagine that she was talking to her kindly old family doctor of years past.

In one of these meditative episodes, the wise old doctor told her that she was bringing it all upon herself. He told her that art school would soon be going better for her, and that she could relax and be kinder to herself for a while. Then he emphatically suggested, "Stop taking all those pills and potions. They just muck up your insides." When Jane shared this with the class, the instructor explained that the information, actually from within herself, was taking the accept-able form of her old family doctor. She was advised to respond as well as she could to what she had learned.

Jane went home and began to scrutinize her behavior in terms of how she might be 'bringing it on herself'. She realized that she tended to eat quickly between classes and art projects, often while talking rapidly to friends. This seemed related to her indigestion difficulties, as she was not chewing thoroughly.

She began to eat more slowly and under calmer circumstances. She learned that this change in her eating speed also resulted in less swallowed air, a major source of digestive system gas. In addition to how she was eating, she began to notice what she was eating. Her diet was largely meat, potatoes, bread, and dairy products. It oc-curred to her that this diet was very low in roughage, thereby adding to her constipation, or possibly even causing it all. She experimented with more fruits, vegetables, and cereals containing bran. Needless to say, her problems began to diminish.

Note that in this case, the absence of medication allowed her inner healing resources maximum efficiency. Without the constipa-tion, the hemorrhoid situation cleared up on its own accord, so that Jane no longer needed refills of the prescription suppositories.

With her new attitude of less worry and tension over school, the headaches diminished dramatically so that she no longer needed the aspirin-codeine combination that she later discovered was a major cause of constipation. Using the meditative technique she had learned, she began to mentally relax instead of taking so many hot baths. Not only did this better relieve her tension, but it relieved the major cause of her itches and rashes - dry skin. In addition, after a long day of sitting doing art work, she began to take walks. This helped her disposition, and the exercise helped her digestion.

This is a clear example of how a person can either be helplessly bewildered or consciously aware. The benefits of awareness over bewilderment are obvious. Listening to an inner directive is a specific technique that can be learned. The guiding source of wisdom may take the form of a kindly old doctor, an ancient medicine woman, a yoga guru, or one's own inner voice describing what is best. The significant message may be expressed in words or in a symbolic image. It may appear during meditation, in a dream or fantasy, or merely pop in to the awareness at an unexpected moment.

Whenever the communication does manifest itself, it is important to realize that one has received intelligent guidance of a very sophisticated sort. Due to an often overly scientific education, many people unfortunately discount messages that do not come from the logical thinking mind. In order to hear and truly respond to one's intuitive flashes, a definite trust is necessary.

Let us now witness how this trust can help bring guidance into the realms of nursing and health care. The following is an example of what it can look like to put more spiritual awareness back into caring:

A patient dying of AIDS in a San Francisco Hospital was near the end stages of his disease process, and had become increasingly belligerent to the staff. Due to the nature of his condition, and to his mental

180

state, no one was eager to work with him. Finally, Jeannette, a staff nurse, agreed to take the assignment.

"First, I went into the laundry room to take a quiet moment. I did some slow, deep breathing, became aware of any feelings and tension in my body, and consciously released them. I prayed and asked for help and guidance in caring for Mr. Smith. I asked to be granted the perfect words and thought to join my soul with him in total harmony, and to be protected from any disease."

"Next," continued Jeannette, "I waited until I felt a peaceful calm envelop me, and I had a vision of an angel hovering near, smiling. I emerged back into the hall, feeling eager to be with Mr. Smith."

"When I entered, he was belligerent initially. When he felt my calm presence, he quieted immediately, and was soon resting. I sat near his bedside, maintaining loving thoughts and sending peaceful energy into the space we shared. His breathing was labored, and I knew he would be leaving the Earth soon. Suddenly, I felt honored to be with him. As if he sensed all this, he then looked up at me and spoke softly."

"I feel so afraid sometimes," he confessed. "It feels like I have the curse, and no one wants to have anything to do with me. I hate to feel like a pariah. It reminds me of my childhood, when I was the last of seven children, and didn't feel welcomed by anyone. No

181

one ever held me or really loved me . . . "

Jeannette said that at that moment, without the least hesitation, she found herself surrounding him in her arms and cradling him like his mother never could. He burst out in deep sobs, and she rocked him for a long tender while. Finally, his sobs subsided gradually, and she felt his body relax and go limp. She had helped usher him to another plane. His peaceful smile and energy let her know that he was fine, and she felt humbled and deeply grateful for the opportunity to share in his transition.

This episode from the life of a nurse helps us all to grasp the countless silent possibilities that exist to share love as people hover between the delicate doorways of birth and death. When nurses can take the time to be with their patients in a deeply caring way, something magical transpires that enables them to substitute in for love never received in times past. Through this tender way of sharing, and lending one's strength, healing can transpire. Healing, in its deepest sense, enriches all participants involved, restoring a sense of balance and harmony.

It is part of my contention, therefore, that a rededication of nursing can only be accomplished through reestablishing the connection between nursing and spirituality. For our inspiration in the modern world, we can look anew at the work of Mother Theresa, often referred to as a modern-day Saint. Her deeply compassionate healing work with the poorest of the poor can motivate us all to look within our hearts and souls. Though we live in a wealthy country, Mother Theresa (who oversees the Sisters of Charity Mission in Harlem) defines ours as a land with a poverty of spirit.

It is my personal observation, after working with and interviewing countless nurses, that many are dying (some literally) to be able to bring their highly spiritual nature back into balance with their overly developed intellectual side. Many nurses, though certainly not all, felt drawn into nursing by what they would term a 'calling', and would be increasingly content with their profession if that deep need within them could be honored. Florence Nightingale herself said that nursing was a calling, not a profession.

Nightingale (as mentioned earlier) also wrote a moving essay in 1852 entitled "Cassandra: Angry Outcry Against the Forced Idleness of Victorian Women". In this work, she shared and transformed her despair about the wasting of women's talents. At the end of this cathartic essay she wrote:

"Awake . . . all ye that sleep, awake." According to Myra Stark, who wrote the introduction to this work, Nightingale felt that the position of women in the nineteenth century was so poor that women of the next century must waken to their power to transform it. Nightingale noted that Christ's great contribution to the advancement of women was to give them a moral existence and relationship to God. "The next Christ," she suggests, "will perhaps be a female Christ."[47] According to Stark, Nightingale considered "Cassandra" as a religious work. Spiritual awareness and dedication gives life a sense of purpose, something missing from the lives of Victorian women, and for this loss of spiritual connection with one's self, and one's purpose, Nightingale lamented.

Waking Up to Oneself

To be guided by inner wisdom, to think and see with the heart, a person must have faith in his or her own deep intelligence. As a

183

culture, however, it seems that we have entirely lost touch with our deepest inner resources. We have lost trust in this form of intuitive knowledge. How has this come to pass?

We have been raised in a society that places enormous overemphasis on that small but loud part of ourselves called the conscious mind. It has become accepted that this logical, thinking consciousness is the autonomous and responsible person, the true self. Actually, the true whole self encompasses much more than our conscious awareness. In fact, the waking consciousness is said to represent only a fraction of the totality of a human being.

Another factor supporting our poor relationship with the inner world is our faith in the external manipulations of technology. Not to dispute the great achievements of science, I merely suggest that one of the effects of this progress has been to allow us the harmful luxury of neglecting a certain degree of responsibility and self-reliance.

Keep in mind, however, that changes in health orientation take considerable time, and it is essential to be kind toward oneself while attempting to adopt a new attitude. The powerful homeostatic tendency is appropriately motivated toward self-preservation. Change must occur slowly and organically to allow for collaboration and adaptation on all dimensions. It is neither possible nor desirable to switch from an externally oriented, non-listening attitude to a meditative, internally directed attitude in a few days. Changes of this magnitude will often take months or even years. One can, nevertheless, begin the process and see where it leads. This may be as simple as taking a class in relaxation or learning meditation techniques.

Caring for one's own health, in the broadest sense, can become a primary interest, a central motivation around which other interests, activities, and relationships are chosen. This new attitude about one's role in their health care can indicate a shift toward a higher level of wellness. One begins to realize that health is the wellspring from which everything else flows, that health offers at least the basic freedom to pursue with optimum energy all that one desires.

This concept is part of nursing's original vision, and one of the most empowering of attitudes. One can continually approach greater health and greater harmony with the world through attention to one's own inner wisdom.

As nurses, it behooves us to remember that a major proponent of this and other holistic concepts was Florence Nightingale. As Dr. Keegan describes in *Holistic Nursing*:

> "The first scientifically trained nurse recognized for her holistic orientation was Florence Nightingale. In her book, *Notes on Nursing* (1859), she shared the essence of her knowledge and wisdom . . . She called attention to the natural antidotes to disease: fresh air, the reparative importance of quiet in the hospital, good lighting, and a properly managed environment . . . She was truly concerned with the body, mind, and spirit of the sick . . . She dared to move beyond the accepted customs of her day, thereby leading her peers, not always with their approval, to higher levels of thinking and performance."[48]

In the words of modern nursing's founder herself, Nightingale said:

> " . . . all disease . . . is more or less a reparative process . . . an effort of nature to remedy a process of poisoning or decay, which has taken place weeks, months,

sometimes years beforehand . . . the symptoms of the sufferings generally considered to be inevitable and incident to the disease are very often not symptoms of the disease at all, but of something quite different - of the want of fresh air, or of light, or of warmth, or of quiet, or of cleanliness, or of punctuality and care in the administration of diet, of each or of all of these . . . The same laws of health or of nursing, for they are in reality the same, obtain among the well as among the sick . . . [49]

Summary

This holistic way of working is our greatest legacy. As nurses, it is up to us to revive the lost art of nursing, that we may know who we are, what our unique contributions are, and how to approach our clients, be they sick or well. It is a great challenge, and one which must be met with dignity, integrity, and clarity. The time is now. We are the chosen ones. Nursing naturally and inherently provides a holistic philosophy with which to meet technology - and to use it wisely.

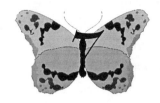

CONSUMER EMPOWERMENT
Conspiring for
Collaborative Care

*It is important that each nurse understand consumer empowerment
and be able to inspire patients in her own way. This chapter shows
nurses how and where to begin empowering patients towards a more
collaborative model of care.*

If we are to make a paradigm shift from a 'sick care system' to
a true 'health care system', changes need to take place within each
component of the system. Consumers are a missing link, an essential
ingredient in the creation of a powerful, effective health care system.
Who could be in a better position to awaken the consumers to their
inner healing potential than empowered nurses? Imagine the example nurses can provide as we become more powerful and creative

as role models.

Health consumers will be able to learn from us how to feel better more of the time. The consumers certainly comprise the largest segment of the system. Therefore, as more and more consumers become less and less 'patient', changing their attitude about their role and expectations for treatment, the entire system will begin to shift.

Together, as a team, providers and consumers can implement changes which will insure that all of our contacts with the health care system are truly healing. First, though, we nurses must inspire this positive forward motion. We need to empower consumers through attitudinal healing, teaching them how to tap into their own inner wisdom, and to learn to trust it in decision making.

Why should we do this? As nurses, we have begun to see ways in which today's medicine can be hazardous to health. We are aware of risks posed by drugs and invasive procedures. We have examined the concept of iatrogenic illness, the unhealthy and often painful (occasionally lethal) results of overly-aggressive medical treatment. We have also seen the financially devastating results of defensive medicine (when doctors overtreat and use unnecessary procedures to protect themselves from possible lawsuits).

In our further examination of modern medical treatment, it has become obvious that one of the most dangerous and disempowering aspects of such aggressive treatment is the increased belief that we (or the patients) have no control over the situation; that people can only become whole again through extensive and expensive medical intervention.

For true healing to occur (for the patients to feel whole, healthy,

190

and released from anguish), they must be empowered to activate *their own* 'inner wisdom' or 'life force'. We have witnessed patients being 'cured', (over and over again), without ever experiencing true and lasting healing. (On the contrary, we have been with patients who died with a deep sense of wholeness and dignity, who felt healed in the face of death.)

When people become participants in their own healing process, they feel powerful, rather than victimized. It is crucial that consumers begin to view themselves differently, to see that they can be the most powerful and essential component in the emerging paradigm.

'Patient' No More: A Manual for the Conscious Consumer

One way consumers can take active control of their health is to assert themselves more. It is important that they understand and acknowledge the true role of nursing, and of the other members of the health team.

Communication with the Nurse

Who could be in a better position to inform clients of health-related issues than the nurse? Yet, what could be more confusing than nursing's present hierarchy? Since its inception in modern times, nursing has been a fragmented group, and it seems the confusion is intensifying.

There is a one-year nurse, a two-year nurse, the diploma graduate (three-year nurse), baccalaureate nurse graduate (four-year nurse), the Clinical Nurse Specialist and the Nurse Practitioner (Masters prepared), and the Ph.D. Nurse. Even nurses have difficulty understanding our stratification, so no wonder the public is confused! For this reason, I will now briefly describe nursing's many categories, so that nurses are clear, and can empower consumers with this basic-level information.

In present-day medical institutions, consumers might anticipate receiving much of their close support and nurturance from nurses, yet it is often the Nurse's Aide or orderly who performs direct primary care. These people help to meet the patient's most basic bodily needs, to keep a supply of linens, snacks, and meals, and can provide an important link between patient and health care professional.

The next person in line is the Licensed Practical Nurse. In today's complex practice, the L.P.N. (or L.V.N.) may represent the feminine principle more than the Registered Nurse. L.P.N.'s receive one year of training, then must pass a licensure examination. Most often, the L.P.N. receives a salary significantly lower than a Registered Nurse, yet is more directly involved in patient care. The duties and privileges of this level of nurse vary from one institution to another, and from state to state.

To me, the name 'practical nurse' seems appropriate and appealing because it implies that the nurse operates on a very basic, practical level. In many ways, nursing should be practical, dealing with the here and now situation, incorporating skills, expertise, and the advantages of any technological innovations available. Many people who wish to become nurses, but are not able to invest the time, energy and finances needed to attend an R.N., program, explore the LPN solution. This role often involves more direct patient

192

care and less opportunity to make nursing judgements.

The two-year nurse has an Associate Degree, usually from a junior or community college. She is eligible to take the exam to be a Registered Nurse, but lacks the advanced education in the arts and sciences that a baccalaureate nurse receives.

The three-year nurse is a vanishing breed. Prior to the last few decades, this was the format for most nurses' 'training', whereby nurses were housed and affiliated with hospitals. They received their clinical education in the hospital setting, and offered a valuable source of assistance to the hospitals. Many diploma schools were associated with colleges, which provided education in the basic sciences. The graduates of this program received a nursing diploma, and were also eligible for the R.N. exam. These nurses had a practical edge in regard to on-the-job experience.

The baccalaureate nurse has completed a four-year program in the university setting, having taken nursing classes, and an array of classes in the arts and sciences, as well as some electives. She is eligible for an R.N. by exam and is awarded a B.S. Degree.

The Clinical Specialist has chosen an area of specialization, and received higher education, at the Master's level in Nursing. She often has to take classes in theory and research, complete a thesis, and becomes a specialist in any one of a variety of clinical areas.

The Nurse Practitioner is also Master's prepared, and trained in diagnosis and treatment of primary and chronic illness. She can provide in-depth health education, performs physical examinations, and can specialize in pediatrics, adult health, women's health, and family practice.

The Ph.D. prepared nurse often functions in nursing education, research, and nursing theory.

According to my standards, a good nurse (at any level) is an open system. She *channels* energy, serving as a link between patient and doctor. In her modern hospital work, she is often called upon to enhance communications between the hospital administration and the physicians. As an example, let me interject a personal story shared by a nurse-client of mine:

"I once achieved the status of Unit Coordinator. What does that mean? What it meant to me by the end of a year is that I was getting paid more than many nurses to take responsibility for some of my colleagues. I had made an agreement to supervise staff and hire and fire as I saw fit to ensure safety and efficiency on my unit."

"What I discovered, however, was that I had a lot of responsibility, with *very* little power. Ultimately, the physicians wielded tremendous power in decision-making within the hospital, but the administration was responsible for the budget. That meant that the doctors had to ask administration for funds, and at times this process resembled a bullfight. Another apt description might be to say it felt like the Tower of Babel, when the people trying to accomplish something all spoke different languages."

"Where was I in the midst of all this? Like a ping pong ball, I was bouncing back and forth between my Unit Administrator and Chief Physician, and also was bouncing back and forth between them and the Hospital

Administrator, who held meetings for Unit Coordinators like me! I scurried from meeting to meeting, trying desperately to keep up with inter-hospital and inner-hospital events. I was sent to Management Development training sessions, and was also responsible for the budget of my unit. In addition to all this, I was also on call to my unit twenty-four hours a day for problems."

This situation, though far from ideal, is typical of the many demands on today's health professionals. In the hierarchy of health team members, each has a different focus and job to do. The person receiving this care can expedite her own process by developing an expanded *awareness.*

For instance, information shared by a patient with a nurse's aide may possibly be transmitted up the ladder, but if the client has an important consideration and wants to be certain it reaches the appropriate persons, the client may need to become more involved. She might need to inquire as to the structure on that particular unit, and as to who is the person in charge. It may, or may not, be sufficient to talk with the overstressed, yet omnipresent manager.

She may even need to write a note or letter to the administration. Many of us who would regularly do this in regard to an unsatisfying service or experience in department stores or other situations, may not even have considered taking this sort of action in hospitals or medical offices. Why is this so?

Perhaps, in medical situations, our fear about our condition, coupled with the high level of financial investment, tends to preoccupy our thoughts. Not only are we not thinking clearly, but we often feel weak and helpless.

Nonetheless, the nurse (theoretically) should be there for the client. Nurses are trained to act on behalf of the patient, and most would prefer to be the patient advocate. I feel it is time for nurses to reclaim this aspect of their work, in order to be more powerful. Nurses can definitely strive to make themselves more available to their patients.

Our clients can be encouraged to communicate with the nurse. All of us, in our various roles in the conspiracy, need to be willing to take risks, to consider that every experience provides us with an opportunity to grow and learn. For example, the client who yells "NURSE!!! Get this slop outta here", will elicit a very different response than the one who says "I could sure use some help when you have a minute".

No one wants to feel inferior or unimportant, and here I refer to consumers and providers alike. Everyone who is dedicated to serving others is able to generate more love and good will when respect for human dignity is maintained. Loss of self-esteem is often followed by a loss of respect from others. For this reason, it is important that consumers learn to maintain their own good feelings of self-love and well-being.

In her workshops for nurses on Therapeutic Touch, Dr. Delores Krieger[50] of N.Y.U. has reminded nurses to take a minute from time to time to 'center'. By this she means to go inward, using the breath to find that place of inner calm. She has advised nurses that even a minute taken in a laundry room (or bathroom stall, if necessary) for inward-directed healing can result in more harmonious interactions. Likewise, there is a much greater likelihood of harmony when the patient, too, attempts to come from a centered place. Nurses can help patients learn centering techniques.

196

Communications with Doctors

Consumers often have plenty of unanswered questions about their care. Many create their own problems by refusing to cooperate with anyone except their doctor. While it is true that the physician makes many of the important decisions about patient care, there are many ways in which the client can participate.

One way the client can become involved is to become more knowledgeable about her condition. The nurse can be an excellent source of health information, especially since she is usually much more accessible. Nurses can remain open to the curiosity of their patients, and can support their assertions toward health.

Clients should be encouraged to remember that nurses, doctors, physical therapists, x-ray technicians, respiratory therapists, etc., are all being affected by the system in which they operate, a force larger than all of us. Consumer empowerment is accelerated when the client takes more and more responsibility for the equality of interactions with all these personnel.

In a book called *How to Choose and Use Your Doctor*, Marvin S. Belsky, M.D.[51] stresses the importance of improving doctor-patient communications. He categorized patients according to their relationship style with their doctor(s), and gives examples based on his practice experience.

Dr. Belsky believes that patients occupy roles based on what they had been taught, and that such roles are either anti-therapeutic or harmful. His categories include:

the ''macho' patient'

the 'I-dare-you-to-find-out-what's-wrong patient'

the 'live-it-up patient'

the 'I-can't-be-bothered patient'

the 'I-need-your-love patient'

the 'you-can't-help-me patient'

the 'cocktail-party patient'

the 'teasing patient'

the 'do-something-for-me patient'

the 'I-can-treat-myself patient'

the 'whip-me patient'

the 'I-don't-want-to-know patient'

He further explains that *fear* is at the root of medical communication problems. The patient puts his fears out, and the physician, in his (perhaps misguided) desire to do something, reassures the patient. The relationship established quickly becomes one of dependency, rather than a partnership aimed at exploring truthful, accurate information.

Here is Dr. Belsky's antidote: The 'smart' patient:

Asks questions

Takes notes

Seeks additional information about her body symptoms, disease

Says what's on his mind

Offers feedback; upsets, feelings, events, ideas, suggestions

Respects his body by health maintenance and restraint

Tries to be an observant, accurate reporter

Shares his experiences with other patients

Doesn't get impatient; recognizes that change takes time

198

Doesn't abdicate responsibility

Welcomes criticism

Leaves his physician for another one when the
relationship is anti-therapeutic

Knows his rights as a patient

Knows his responsibilities as a patient

Trusts his feelings, and his ability to make judgements[53]

Finally, to conclude our discussion about doctor-patient relationships, consider that the wise use of physicians as a medical resource requires forethought on several questions:

1. What is bothering me and what do I really want to do
   about it?

2. Do I really need help with it?

3. Have I considered which type of doctor (or health
   practitioner) would be most helpful? A properly
   chosen specialist whose personality suits me can save
   time, heartache, and money.

4. Am I being realistic about the help I want?
   Patients sometimes demand the impossible. Doctors
   are merely other people with technical expertise and
   knowledge. Freedom from all human ills and suffering
   is not within their power to give. Neither are
   accurate life expectancy predictions within the
   doctors' power to give.

5. How can I make it easy for the doctor to help me?

6. Are their any attitudes on my part (anger, mistrust, etc.) that will diminish the quality of services I receive?

Remember, better communications with our doctors would help improve the quality not only of our own treatment, but of the whole system.

Communications with Ancillary Staff

A great variety of technical experts exist within the walls of medical facilities and institutions. Some, such as respiratory therapists, physical therapists, and pharmacists, have spent many years pursuing the specialized knowledge of their own field. Others, such as laboratory technicians, ward clerks, and x-ray and EKG assistants have received special training of often shorter duration, and are generally supervised by medical specialists.

In order to receive the best care from all of these categories, it remains crucial for the client to be clear in communications, respectful, and willing to persevere towards achieving his own personal health goals. A most effective way to accomplish this is through a friendly and cordial acknowledgment of each person's unique contributions.

Communication with the Body

In considering ways in which the health care consumer can become more powerful, we must examine the beliefs consumers have held about their bodies. As has been mentioned, the present medical

200

system has been based on a fear-provoking foundation. Patients are encouraged to do or not to do certain treatments by instilling a negative image ("if you don't do this, you'll die from a disease").

Since we are a death-denying culture, much of this fear is compounded by our cultural fears. In other parts of the world, people have more intimate contact with death, and view death as an inevitable part of life, sometimes even an event to be celebrated. In our culture, with its enormous emphasis on youth, we relegate the aging and the dying to long-term care facilities, where they are no longer visible in the mainstream of daily life.

Health care consumers have learned to dread disease, and to despise the physical evidence of the aging process. From an early age, we tend as a culture to neglect the body and its needs as much as possible, considering this attitude to be one of strength. There is much denial surrounding the body in general, and particularly as regards the signals from our body which often precede disease. Were we each to learn about the ways in which our body supports us, we would not need to fear its messages. When we deny their meaning, we compound illness.

The body speaks. It has sophisticated forms of communication. In our amazing interconnections, we have innate mechanisms which relay information from one body system to another. The chemical neurotransmitters send messages along the nervous system to the brain, which relays information and responses back to the source. We are truly miraculous beings, with highly developed abilities to learn about and respond to the call of discomfort long before it develops into dis-ease.

Take, for example, the case of Maria, a nurse working on a coronary care unit. She was sixty pounds overweight, smoked, and

201

had a family history of heart disease. In Caryn Summers' book, *Caregiver, Caretaker*, she mentions that often nurses choose fields to work in that somehow have a personal meaning in their lives. She calls this syndrome 'the chase', whereby the person creates a subtle reenactment of her fears, an attempt to heal an early drama through reliving it.

For Maria, her father (a chain smoker), died suddenly of a heart attack when she was a child, and later her mother developed coronary disease and had several operations. Maria vowed to try to do something to stop this deadly killer, so there she was, working furiously in her cardiac unit to try to feel less powerless.

What is wrong with this picture? The problem I see is that Maria's intent is in the right place, but she has not paid attention to the clues. The dietary habits she learned at an early age have obviously contributed to her obesity, the addiction to smoking has further compromised her abilities to defend herself against familial disease patterns, and most importantly, *she is conveying a very mixed message to her patients.* How can she possibly, in good faith, counsel them against heart disease when she is obviously placing herself at such high risk?

As has been mentioned at great length, for nurses to create a new image for ourselves, we have to make some obvious changes. Just as it has been hard to believe the fat doctor who smokes when he tells us that smoking is bad for us, so is it ludicrous for nurses to try to be counselling people about health issues (which is what our licensure grants us power to do), without first becoming living examples.

The old adage "do as I say, not as I do" has always seemed absurd to us, even as children. The truth is that we do watch other people's behavior to learn about life. The struggling young business-man looks to his supervisors to show him how to do it, just as new nurses look to the more 'seasoned' professionals to model the way. Whether we like it or not, we are always speaking loudly with our actions.

In examining styles of communication, it is important to consider the concept of 'inauthentic communication'. When a person tells us something, if we are paying attention we will often notice that we have a visceral response to their words. Sometimes that response is a reaction to the way they have relayed the message (for example, "GET THOSE SHOES OUT OF HERE OR I'LL BREAK YOUR NECK" will certainly draw a different response than if someone leans over and gently whispers in your ear *"I love you, and think you're the most wonderful person alive. Could you please put your shoes elsewhere?"*)

However, if a person says "I really like your new haircut" (trying to be nice), but in their heart they are really thinking "That is the stupidest thing she's ever done; I can't wait till Shirley sees it; she'll die laughing", usually the person receiving the statement can perceive that something is out of line; that somehow her words are not ringing true. This is an example of inauthentic communication, where the feelings and words don't match.

Another example is the proverbial person who is banging the desk, red-faced, and screaming, "I AM NOT ANGRY! I NEVER GET ANGRY!" In this example, the person's words do not match their actions. People who receive mixed messages like this almost always end up with some degree of confusion. That is because the person who spoke the message is not being honest, even with herself. Inauthentic communication is another example of how denial serves

203

to keep us from the truth about a situation.

In order to inspire health consumers to take affirmative action on their own behalf, we nurses are now coming face to face with our own challenges. We are being asked to 'clean up our act', to be willing to squarely face our own addictions, and to overcome the compulsive behaviors that are largely a result of our own denial.

Once we are in honest integrity with ourselves, and not lying about our lives, needs, or habits, we will be thoroughly believable as role models for a challenging, yet exhilarating, process of freeing ourselves from the tyranny of denial. Then we will be in a perfect position to teach consumers (and doctors!) about this process, from our own first-hand experiences.

Our bodies are designed to communicate with us in a variety of ways. People have feelings, visions, dreams, hopes, aspirations, and pain. Each of these represents another way in which our inner world is trying to make contact with our outer world, since we humans are multi-faceted beings.

In *The Prophet,* a well-known inspirational book of ancient wisdom, Kahlil Gibran speaks of the concept of pain:

> Your pain is the breaking of the shell that encloses
>   your understanding
> Even as the stone of the fruit must break, that its heart
>   may stand in the sun
> So must you know pain . . .
> And could you keep your heart in wonder at the daily
>   miracles of your life
> Your pain would not seem less wondrous than your
>   joy; and you would accept the seasons of your heart,

204

even as you have always accepted the seasons
  that pass over your fields.
And you would watch with serenity through the
  winters of your grief.
Much of your pain is self-chosen.
It is the bitter potion by which the physician within
  you heals your sick self.
Therefore trust the physician, and drink his remedy in
  silence and tranquility;
For his hand, though heavy and hard, is guided by the
  tender hand of the Unseen,
And the cup he brings, though it burn your lips, has
  been fashioned of the clay which the Potter has
  moistened with his own sacred tears.[54]

Putting Ourselves in Our Own Hands

How can we learn to start paying attention to the body's 'words'?
There are several processes that teach health care consumers more
about this kind of communication. To determine more of our body's
needs, we can resort to our powers of *deduction, meditation, integration, and experimentation.*

In deduction, we can use our reasoning ability to arrive at a
logical conclusion based on the evidence provided, similar to the
way we solve mysteries or win competitive games. In our daily lives,
clues are often being offered about our state of well-being or dis-ease
(remember, this word refers to a state of discomfort; it does not have
to progress to illness if heeded early). Ultimately, one can remember

to use powers of deduction to achieve higher levels of wellness by following the clues. Considering the 'health game' in this manner can make it much more fun to become and stay healthy.

We can also use our powers of meditation, whereby we journey inward to consult with our inner guidance. In a fascinating book called *The Master Game*,[55] it is suggested by Robert S. De Ropp that for most of us, the inner world remains a vast and vague territory. According to De Ropp, our ability to achieve awakening (and thus health) depends upon our acceptance of this statement: ". . . man's ordinary state of consciousness, his so-called waking state, is not the highest level of consciousness of which he is capable." Higher levels are available through inner exploration.

Other similar experts remind us that we need to be clear that the information we receive outwardly is harmonious with the information from our deep inner voice. Certainly, were more of us to remember this, we would not do things we didn't feel right about, and not live with so many regrets.

In the process of integration, we allow the parts to assemble in our mind in order to conjure up an image of the whole, for example, if we become aware of pain in some body part, then we may wish to notice if there are any other aches or symptoms. Our end goal is to put the pieces of the puzzle together into a coherent picture.

When we consider the word 'healing', we see that it comes from the Greek root word 'halos', meaning 'whole, hale, hearty'. The word 'holy' is also derived from the same word. According to the ancient tradition of homeopathy, healing occurs from the inside out, and from top to bottom. Ultimately, the inside and outside must meet in a unified whole.

We can choose to view ourselves as energy systems, and devote ourselves to the integration of all our components. Is there a connection between the pain in another area and this painful spot? Is there a relationship between recent activities and the feelings I have now? Taking charge of our health in this manner is not only empowering, it is *fun*!

We can also use experimentation to learn to meet our physical needs. To do this, we choose to use the body as a laboratory. In Eastern philosophy, the body is considered to be the temple for the spirit. If the walls of the temple began to show evidence of cracking, would not wise people examine the foundation? Would they not also consider what is going on inside the edifice? If they were to discover that inner activities were responsible for the cracks, would it not make sense to change the actions that resulted in destruction of the temple?

After these changes were made, how would the people evaluate whether their actions were successful? They would keep a close watch on the temple walls. If they were unable to ameliorate the destructive condition from an internal approach, they would likely resort to external manipulations, first locally, then even altering conditions further away.

Similarly, we can pay attention to our bodies to see if the actions we choose to take are supportive to our 'temple'. We can experiment to ascertain what situations are contributing to our state of dis-ease by trying various internal manipulations. If, after a reasonable amount of experimentation, we did not feel successful, we could try a more external approach, which ultimately could include environmental changes.

Environmental health is a nursing issue! Each person has the opportunity to become political in terms of environmental watch; we are all affected by the external environment in which we exist. Nurses, as guardians of the health and public welfare, must become more environmentally aware and active.

Many people take more responsibility for the care of their cars than the care of their own bodies. We listen carefully and ask a multitude of questions when our car is being diagnosed, yet how many people maintain the attitude "Here's my body, Doc. What time shall I pick it up?"

Learning to pay attention to your body's language can save you years of pursuing other people's fears. Learning to experiment with the body can give information no matter what you do, for if what you try does not work, sometimes it will cause an exacerbation in the symptoms, which also gives you valuable information.

Consumer Self-Advocacy

Some say that according to the laws of nature, we get as many lessons as we need. Unless you make a needed change, the pain will arise as many times, and in as much intensity, as is necessary to get the message across. It is healing, therefore, to learn to pay careful attention to our bodies. We can consider that our body is the message carrier from our internal to our external world.

Changes that occur on the body level are accompanied by more subtle changes on the mental or spiritual level. For example, making healthier food choices can quickly affect family relationships or job efficiency.

George Ohsawa, a world reknowned expert on macrobiotic

208

theory, commented that our Western medicine is severely handicapped due to its belief that we can not change our body cells simply by taking in the proper nutrients. "Such a concept eliminates a connection between foods, cells, organs, body, and mind. This is the most important shortcoming of modern medicine."[56]

Think about the misconceptions many of us carry to the present day concerning illness. Can you imagine how your life (and that of your patients) might be different if, when young, someone told you the following: "The only time you will get sick is if you ignore the gentle calls from within your own body. What will happen is that more body parts will join together to get your attention, and then you must devote even *more* energy to your self. It will serve you well to listen closely when your body speaks."

Many present day health experts have praised the benefits of movement therapies. One of these was Moshe Feldenkrais.[57] Concentrating on the relationship between the nervous and muscular systems, he believed that as we train our bodies to achieve the various forms of which it is capable, our self-image is enhanced and we increase in strength and flexibility.

Where does this process begin? Is it too late to start conditioning our bodies at a later stage of our lives? For those who have remained current on the research related to heart attacks and exercise, we know that strengthening one's physical body is a continual process. Today can be a great time to tone up a little more than we did yesterday, and a little less than we will do tomorrow. As time passes, we find that what once stressed our bodies immensely is now something we can accomplish with ease. Often it takes less time to build up endurance than we first imagine when we take note of our physical status.

We need to keep in mind that the body is amazingly resilient. What happens frequently is that we forget where the 'buttons' are to release tension (or energy) in the body. Hans Selye, world-reknowned expert on stress, agrees that healthy minds reside in healthy bodies. He suggests that we find and use the particular mental and physical buttons that fit our own personal situations.

Alexander Lowen[58], bioenergetics expert, talks about how the healthy person enjoys spontaneity and an enhanced sense of freedom. Bioenergetics theory stresses the importance of *breathing*. Most of us tend to breathe rather shallowly, particularly when we are in a state of fear or anxiety. Our chest muscles tighten. For this reason alone, regular exercise and movement can support our state of relaxation and well-being. As the body becomes more flexible through movement, the mind expands to accommodate the increased energy.

When considering where to begin adding exercise into your daily life, it is important to start where it feels right to you - for you - taking into account all your physical, psychological, and financial demands. For many people, running is blissful and effortless. For others, it is pure torture.

To ascertain which exercise suits you best, you must be willing to engage in active experimentation. Try a form, and perform it for a trial period. If it does not feel good, let it go. There are many forms of exercise, from aerobic dancing to calisthenics, from martial arts (Aikido, Judo, Tai chi) to yoga. Some people prefer fast physical exercise at times. At other times, they enjoy a slower approach, like yoga or Tai chi, which blends spiritual practices with physical exercise.

Any place is a good place to start, for there may be as many paths toward well-being and optimal health as there are people.

210

Continue to learn about yourself, and what works best for you, and be nourished in your growth.

Movement As Self-Therapy

As a personal example, I loved to dance and do acrobatics as a child. My life changed when I tore the cartilage in my knee at age twelve. From then on, I was advised to be very careful, which definitely crimped my style. A few years later, I tore the cartilage in my other knee while performing gymnastics, and in my senior year of high school I had surgery when the first knee swelled and tore again. I was told by the doctors that I would never dance again, and that if I wasn't very careful, I would require surgery on my other knee as well.

For well over twenty years, I gave up the dream of being a dancer. Dance had always provided an outlet for me, a place to breathe heavily, to be creative and graceful, and to release emotional anguish. In giving up dance I gave up a large part of the magic in my life.

Then four years ago my oldest daughter, who was nine at the time, asked me to take her to a bellydance class. She had watched the bellydancers at a local festival, and loved the beautiful graceful movements. I was then forty years old, slightly overweight and out of shape after my third birth. I had planned to sit along the sidelines and watch the class, but the instructor would not hear of it. She encouraged me to get up and get moving.

Gingerly, I imitated her movements, watching my misshapen body struggle to emulate the smooth gyrations. It brought up a lot of

211

feelings for me, as I used to look so strong and powerful, and now felt soft and mushy. As it turned out, I decided to join my daughter regularly, since the class provided a space for us to be together and share something special. I loved the comeraderie of women after feeling 'stuck at home' for ten years.

I felt nurtured and supported in this environment, and after only a few weeks, a different woman was peeking back at me in the mirror! She was graceful, and curvaceous. I began to remember who I really was, having lost myself to the constant demands of a decade of motherhood. I felt renewed and rejuvenated, and the extra pounds began to slip away as I wiggled and writhed in front of the mirror.

Today, I have been bellydancing for four years, and my life has changed dramatically. I am at the perfect weight for my body, I love the way I look and feel, and I am convinced that this movement form is ancient female medicine. I have found beautiful books to support this belief.[59]

We nurses especially need to reclaim our bodies and our strength. We may need some 'special medicine' to get back on track in our work. From my point of view, bellydance coupled with emotional release is a perfect combination. You may wish to experience this combination (I use it in my healing retreats), or create your own healing rituals, and encourage your clients to do the same.

Consumer Tools: Personal Survival Kit

There are many ancient and modern tools for healing. In some systems of analysis, such as Oriental Diagnosis, Hand Analysis, Astrology, and Personology (body structure analysis), our body types and temperaments are linked. Theoretically, we can change them through conscious effort. These changes can be effected through a change in *diet, attitude, exercise, and awareness.* As the inner self goes through changes (i.e., perhaps I finally accept my 'undesirable' physical characteristics, no longer devoting precious energy to changing or disliking parts of myself), the energy flow increases in other areas of my life.

In this manner, the 'upward spiral' has begun. We begin to feel better and better because we are taking more and more positive action. As our creative energies continue to spark, we are being transformed. Our entire being will reflect these changes in lifestyle, for no longer are we tense, disappointed, or dissatisfied. We feel better, we are much more relaxed, our capillaries and muscles are relaxed.

The more relaxed we remain, the more energy our body has at its disposal to devote towards healing and regeneration. As more time is spent in restful, regenerative activities, we begin to look different. An example of this occurs when we take, at long last, a much-needed vacation. 'How wonderful you look' . . .Surely we feel better every time someone tells us this, so it becomes self-fulfilling prophecy.

As we incorporate various tools to relax and support our bodies (don't forget the tremendous value of *massage*, which relaxes our muscles and allows the blood to flow better), we find ourselves changing our habits and lifestyles. These changes can become a permanent part of us, so that we begin to appear rested and feel ready to meet life's challenges more of the time.

As we keep our joints mobile with regular stretching, as we keep our hands limber, and our body active, our minds open. The

213

mind, as you may recall, channels energy. Often, those who have open minds are more flexible in their lives. These people appear young, even with physical evidence of ageing. Conversely, it would be difficult to be especially rigid in thought when you are quite flexible in body. The power of concentration necessary to do such movements as are performed in yoga, for example, is gained by redirecting one's thoughts inward, excluding the great distractor, mind-chatter. Anytime we can stop our thoughts from ruling us, our bodies benefit.

Thus, we have established that the attitudes of a consumer are reflected in her inner health. Conversely, we see that if she achieves a state of inner peace and harmony, she'll feel better on the outside as well.

It is now crucial that the 'patient' *stop being patient* and instead become a responsible and active consumer, one who seeks harmony and balance in her life. It may serve us well to cease calling them 'patients', lest the term become a self-fulfilling prophecy. There are many changes needed, and perhaps they have been 'patient' for far too long.

It is time to examine our medical belief system, using the very tools we have just discussed. When we stop the mind-chatter, using meditation or some other form of inner-directed search, we can hear the inner voice that will guide us most clearly towards health and wholeness. Rather than become fearful when signs of dis-ease approach, we can use our awareness to restore well-being.

It is not easy, however, for most of us to snap our fingers and say "O.K. now I'm in a state of inner peace and harmony". It is often a gradual process that requires changes in personal and cultural attitudes. As I see it, there are three major attitudes that directly

214

affect our level of physical well-being.

Self-Love, Open-Mindedness, and Self-Responsibility

In learning to change some of our unhealthy attitudes, we might need to reprogram our unwillingness to love and care for ourselves. Our culture often labels self-caring as selfishness. *Self-love*, in a health-related definition, involves being willing to trust our own inner wisdom as well as the trained wisdom of health professionals. Listening to inner guidance is an act of power and self-love.

In looking at the concept of self-love as related to healing, we can look to the words of Erich Fromm, who wrote the well-known classic *The Art of Loving.*[60] In this book, Dr. Fromm examines Western thought concerning self-love, and explains that it has often been viewed as a negative trait, that the person loves himself to the exclusion of loving others (which is, in reality, an extreme case). Fromm states: "The affirmation of one's own life, happiness, growth, and freedom is rooted in one's capacity to love . . . If an individual is able to love productivity, he loves himself, too . . ."[61]

One of the ways we express self-love is the care we give to our physical selves. It takes many of us years, if not a lifetime, to learn the special language of our own bodies. We often forget to spend time with ourselves, finding out what we need. We jump from one costume to another as we change roles, often neglecting to acknowledge the body. We seek lovers to caress and stroke us, neglecting to consider how much love we could give to ourselves. Those who seek love through sexuality alone generally find themselves unable to

215

love fully with the heart.

Open-mindedness involves learning to take responsibility for one's own health while simultaneously unlearning the 'victim role' of the patient. Asserting your inner wisdom is every bit as important as having it, and it is the next logical step in the process towards self-love and self-trust.

Too often people are willing to blindly accept what they are told, without listening to the voice within. The doctor tells them something; they have further information that may make a difference in his response, but it seems too burdensome to mention. Stop!! Look at this process. This is one of the ways we disempower ourselves. This is how we cheat ourselves out of the best information that medical science has to offer. Take the time. Risk feeling foolish. The stakes are too high to do otherwise.

Open-mindedness also relates to changing our ideas about certain aspects of our lives. A wise physician-friend of mine had a statue in his office. It was a knight in a suit of armor, about ten inches tall. Pierced through his sword was a tiny piece of notebook paper on which was scrawled the message, "the secret of life is not to do what you like, but to like what you do". The image of the suit of armor seems apt, for often we are so stuck in our 'armor' that we forget the value of letting in new information.

People who assume *self-responsibility* feel joyous and more self-confident. It seems that one reason for this is that they are significantly less subject to the ill effects of their fears. Knowing more about our bodies enable us to open up the infinite possibilities from which we can choose. We can venture further from the beaten path, secure within ourselves that we are strong, capable beings equipped with the skills for survival.

216

We have much to learn, and we also have much to unlearn. We are amazingly intricate machines, with many interdependent systems, all of which must be functioning maximally for us to achieve a high level of wellness. *The greatest danger to your health is to give away responsibility for it!* The hardest part of healing one's self is to replace the dependency on doctors and drugs with a new reliance on inner wisdom and intuition. Yet this is the medicine that is required.

Enhancing Self-Awareness and Recovery

We have much to unlearn because our institutions of learning have often been closed-minded. We have not provided our children with useful, open-minded information about their bodies. We have not chosen to insist, as health educators and parents, that our schools take responsibility for teaching children some of the most important information they will need to survive as healthy adults. According to the well-known phrase of social scientist Ashley Montague,[62] "We die intellectually and spiritually by 'degrees'." His emphasis was on the lack of appreciation for uniqueness and creativity in our institutions of higher learning.

Nursing education, for example, has not always promoted the growth of the participants. Often, a standardization and stifling of individual creativity has been encouraged to facilitate the mechanical operation. We all know it takes courage to be different, and that life can seem to be more unstable and insecure as we abandon our rigid beliefs and open up to new information.

It is often more difficult to unlearn something than to learn something new. We have been taught not to rely on our self-healing

217

abilities. Taking responsibility for our bodies means unlearning.

Primarily, we must unlearn that only physicians are responsible for our health and well-being. The media continue to refer to the major killers (diseases) as if they were bolts of lightning striking only innocent victims. As we have seen, we can avoid certain diseases by improving our health habits and building immunity.

The process for recovery, therefore, is four-fold. First, we must acknowledge having given our power away. Second, we need to make a conscious decision to re-own our power. Third, we need to strengthen our physical/emotional body with loving care. Fourth, we can strengthen our spiritual self with food for the soul.

What could be food for the soul? For some, like myself, it is dance. For others, it is music, or art. For some, it can be massage, or visualization. At times, it can be reading, meditation, or sexual contact. The ways to uplift the spirit are many.

Once again, according to John Bradshaw, the well-known codependency expert, affirmations are food for the soul. Affirmations are positive statements that affirm the good about us, and in our lives. "I am a strong and powerful healer"; "I am loved and honored by all those I hold in high regard"; "I am happy and healthy". Saying the words is not enough to effect powerful changes, for sometimes we are in denial about our truest beliefs. It is important that we believe the positive affirmations, and learn to eliminate our negative self-fulfilling prophecies.

In making healthy changes, it is crucial to feel good about ourselves, and to come from a position of strength. This can be a most difficult challenge when we are ill, for we are bombarded with negative feelings, which eventually lead to a lack of self-love. To

218

change these feelings, we must develop the final ingredient for high-level wellness, faith.

Converting Fear into Faith

As we find ourselves plummeting into a negative spiral, we need to reach deep within ourselves to that place where we have stored our faith. Many people profess to have little or no faith, yet when faced with crisis, they find themselves reaching inward to find that well-spring of comfort.

Some spiritual teachers consider *faith* to be the flip side of *fear*. Fear can be viewed as the perpetuation of negative thought patterns which can eventually manifest in our reality, particularly as we give them more energy. Each of us must learn to manage our fears in order to live fully and experience the moment. When we learn to embrace our fears, yet not to give them power over us, we have begun our journey towards empowerment.

Fear is the foundation of our entire medical system today. We are bombarded with negative messages about our bodies, and our ability to effect change within ourselves, and when we believe that we are 'powerless' or 'victims' to dis-ease, we have allowed fear to control us. Eliminating the roots of our bodily-related fears can put each of us in the drivers seat, allowing ourselves to accept gentle guidance, honoring our knowledge and love of self in the decision-making process.

Here is how fears manifest themselves on the physical plane. I am afraid to do something . . . I picture myself undergoing physical and/or emotional trauma and anguish. This picture becomes part of

219

me in several ways. I may create the dreaded situation in my unconscious efforts to face the fear. This encounter can take the form of a dream, or actual incident.

I may also store the fear in my body, where it emerges time and again on various levels to haunt me. If I do not deal with the fear, or confront it, it can intensify and have power over me. The fear, in actuality, is nothing more than energy, stored in the form of emotion. By ignoring the fear, the emotions may seem to subside, but the energy is blocked, and builds. A blockage, in any form, impedes our abilities to run energy through ourselves.

Fear is, therefore, a channeling of energy in a certain form. *Faith* is also a channeling of energy in another form. Our fears are often a result of our need to protect certain belief systems. Whereas one person may interpret a situation as pleasant and harmonious, another may face the exact same experience with dread and fear. We often create our realities, so our most healthy response might be to learn from our friends how to feel better about the situation, and transform our fear into faith.

A patient's faith, alone, can bring about amazing changes in physiological function. It is certainly in our power to be aware of the need to turn our fears into faith (that the right thing will happen; that we are protected), and to approach issues of health and wellness with a sense of personal power.

Tap the Source of Boundless Energy

All of these concepts have been based on a simple understanding of 'energy'. Though perhaps difficult to define, every healer *knows* energy, *feels* energy, and has learned to work with it. Energy is what we are; all living things are energy systems within larger energy systems. Good health and smooth functioning represent an unimpeded flow of energy, while illness represents a block.

To thoroughly explore the concept of how our mind sets our reality into action, consider this health-related example:

Suppose that we are receiving a message from deep within ourselves (i.e., we can't seem to relax because we owe money on our credit cards, and we want to be able to relax). Suddenly, we are stuck in deep, obsessive thought about this issue.

There are many ways to deal with this situation, and the outcomes would vary depending upon the choices we make. We may choose to continue on in our belief that we can't relax, and if so, chances are good that we will remain tense, and therefore less healthy.

We may also, however, take one of the numerous choices available, such as to dip into our savings, or work overtime, or sell something we own that may alleviate the strain, or even consider writing a letter to the credit card company explaining our circumstances and soliciting their aid in the process. Each of these actions would invite different circumstances to develop. We may not always get the desired response, but that which we have set into motion by our thought-seed creates a new reality to be dealt with.

If the choice is to ignore the nagging inner voice, we may develop physical symptoms, such as an ulcer or heart attack, or mental ones, such as depression and anxiety. Sometimes our resistance is lowered, and we get less drastic irritations; eczema, for example, or asthma, or boils.

An alternative choice would be to acknowledge the stressor (in

221

this case financial) and meditate on it. It would be like consulting your inner accountant, the one who has been scheming all along. Determine what your goal was in having handled matters this way, and ascertain whether it is time to reevaluate the approach. Your meditation may serve to demonstrate that you can create some distance between yourself and what you perceive of as your 'problem', hence gaining a new perspective. In the end, you may choose not to alter the situation at this time, and make a conscious decision not to expend any more energy (in the form of worry) on this topic.

In meditation, we 'shed some light' on the topic, and are more able to see options from which to choose. Knowing that we have the ability to do this allows us some relaxation, since we instantly feel less helpless. By concentrating, we are more able to gain some clarity and see that perhaps the real problem is not the money, per se, but rather how we have chosen (consciously or unconsciously) to deal with it.

Many of us may concentrate on money, and through our intense efforts, we may succeed in drawing it to us. But if we still do not feel good, we may need to change our orientation. When we define our priorities with crystal clarity, we affect the entire chain of events that make up our lives. If we focus on our health as a top priority, it is likely that the rest of our lives will work effectively.

Meanwhile, we are enjoying ourselves so much in the process that we can not help but to attract life-supporting experiences. With this positive quality to our daily lives, we are each well on our way to making our special contribution towards upgrading the quality of life on this planet. This is, in its highest sense, the fulfillment of the positive concept of conspiracy.

Maslow's hierarchy states that when all of our energy is devoted to physical survival, we have a difficult time reaching our dreams, or loftier ideals. If this is true, perhaps we would all benefit from concentrating on staying well and feeling healthy, and considering this a basic goal. If we were to insist that we were well more of the time, we could free up other energy for the things that we really want to create in our lives. This is exactly how we turn the situation around, into an upward spiral.

Have we not all known people who seem to be 'kissed by the blarney stone'? Or others, like PigPen in the Peanuts character strip, who are always in the middle of a mess? It is easy to blame our lives on 'luck', and much more difficult to gain an awareness of our role in its creation. It is also difficult to teach this concept, because those who have great difficulty are often so wrapped up in their ill fortune that they perpetuate the downward motion of the spiral without knowing that they have a part in it.

For this very reason, illness can be seen as a blessing in disguise. The normal circuitry within the body is interrupted, so the energies won't flow, and in some way the body shuts down. It seems to be a strong communication; "Alright, buddy, that does it! I'm going on strike . . ." and the next thing we know, we are watching the world go by from a horizontal plane. Often, however, this is *exactly* the medicine that is needed, and we heal with nothing more than a rest to promote proper energetic balancing.

Emotional Release As A Turning Point

Let us consider other possibilities. The person has emotions which need to be experienced or somehow integrated. Generally, we have been taught to experience our 'positive' emotions, while suppressing those we enjoy less, are uncomfortable with, or which are socially less acceptable. This very act of blocking energy, including our pain, causes a surplus build-up in the body. As the pressure continues to mount in certain areas, most often in the weakest of our organs or systems, we begin to feel a call from the affected area.

If it were expressed in English, it might be saying, "yoohoo, you up there . . .remember me???", and we look down, startled at times, that there are actual physical changes. Our body may have been gently nudging us for quite a while before screaming for attention in this manner. Alas, we often wander in our lives onto loftier ideals, neglecting the importance of the physical plane. The laws of nature unfold, and survival of the fittest occurs on the bodily level, the inevitable result being the collapse of our weakest link. We are then called upon for a very important mission - time to heal the body.

Those who, on the other hand, remain in such close communication with their bodies that they are aware of even the most subtle messages, do not wait for illness or shut-down. Instead, they initiate the necessary lifestyle changes immediately. When we are not in close contact with our body, or when we are in denial, we are drawn back to reality through bodily 'screams'. This is what we call, in medical terms, a crisis.

Webster defines *crisis* as *the turning point for better or worse*. Most of us tend to emphasize the negative aspects of crisis, and overlook the possibility that things might change for the better through this experience. Emergency scenes are difficult and traumatic, yet they teach us lessons. As nurses, it is important for us to recall that hospitalization can be the perfect turning point for our patients.

Years ago, sanatoriums were popular. These provided a very different atmosphere from our modern hospitals. The sanatorium was a health resort to which well-known personalities 'resorted' for rest and tranquility between periods of great duress.

Today, people in high positions tend to operate chronically under enormous stress, without acknowledging the need for rest and regeneration. This pattern is directly related to our cultural denial, and refusal to honestly admit our human vulnerabilities.

This syndrome has greatly contributed to the enormous amount of chronic disease in our society, everything from cancer to 'Chronic Fatigue Syndrome' (even the Creator took a day of rest after working for six!). People who are debilitated by this modern disease of our times have to rest 18-20 hours a day, and are often people who have pushed themselves beyond their bodily warnings and endurance for years. These people are then 'given' the opportunity, by their own body, to take a break from their 'normal' existence and reflect upon their lives.

Moments of illumination often come when the mind is still. Though the thought of trying to still the mind during crisis appears difficult, we only need to experience this phenomenon during less acute times to recognize the value of these quiet moments of inner harmony. Often, as soon as we devote energy to inner peace, our vision crystallizes into clear thought.

Moments of such crystal-clear vision in a hospital setting are rather limited, particularly for the patient. Imagine that you are a patient in a hospital, and are suddenly blessed with a more relaxed consciousness. You may have done a meditation, or dozed, to awaken and realize that this illness is exactly what you have needed all along. You begin to appreciate the gift of your situation, and abandon the fear you were carrying. Now you know why you're there, and can see the light at the end of a previously dark tunnel. With this new

225

awareness, you can peacefully meet the pain, and devote yourself to the intriguing task of learning to decipher the body message and take appropriate action.

However, a stigma of guilt seems to be attached to restful periods in modern living. How many times have you heard people justify their need for vacation ("I had to get away - I was going crazy!" or "I needed to sit down for a few minutes - my feet were killing me!").

As nurses, it seems we are subject to this same misguided thinking, and often work double shifts without allowing ourselves to rest and regenerate afterwards. This behavior and attitude contributes to nursing's high degree of 'burnout'. We can only go so long without recharging our batteries, and the sooner we nurses get real and honest with ourselves, the sooner we will provide a source of modeling and inspiration to health care consumers.

Summary and Invitation to Join the Conspiracy:

How nurses can inspire their clients to 'conspire':

1. Start by showing them, through your actions and words, how to assert themselves in a healthy manner. Insist on more humane treatment for both consumers and providers.

Explain to them that nurses have been trying to speak up for years, but we have been too enmeshed in hospital machinery to speak clearly. Many of us have lost our positions for being outspoken.

Nursing desperately needs the support of informed consumers, who are willing to risk the irritated stares of a physician or hospital administrator. Not everyone can be verbal. Many of our patients are too weak, mentally or physically, to become involved on this level. For this reason, those who are able to speak out must.

Teach them to ask about procedures. Have clients be willing to ask if they're *really* necessary. Support their willingness to ask questions until they are satisfied with the answers. If a person is not convinced that a procedure is absolutely necessary, maybe he or she should not have it. It is, after all, their body, their life, and their choice!

It is up to each of us to help restrain runaway technology, and to ensure that hospitals are safe, compassionate places for people to heal. We can each start wherever we find ourselves, whenever a situation gives us cause for reflection. Whenever something seems uncomfortable, unhealthy, or unnecessary, that is a place for us to assert ourselves.

As a simple example, hospitals are filled with limited spectrum fluorescent lighting. How many of you have noticed feeling weird when under these lights? I personally get a headache and feel agitated after minutes of constant, low-level flickering and buzzing. These can be replaced by quieter, full-spectrum tubes, which are much more natural and tranquilizing for the human system.

Do consumers expect the hospitals to replace these irritants just because one, or many, nurses suggest it? It will not happen. Hospitals will change when consumers - who pay the bills - insist upon healthy changes.

There are also a lot of odors and germs in hospital settings and clinics. If enough patients or family insisted on fresh air, uncontaminated drinking water, and real food, it would change (how

227

could they still be serving jello, with lots of sugar and extremely low nutritional food value and artificial dyes that could possibly be carcinogenic?). Florence Nightingale insisted on ventilating hospitals properly, and increasing hygienic conditions. Now we must all conspire to assure ourselves healthy working and recuperating conditions today.

2. Learn to overcome fears and move into powerful action.

The medical system is tied up in knots of confusion. Fear, finance, and runaway technology are overshadowing common sense and compassion. If doctors function with enormous amounts of fear, do the nurses and consumers have to buy into this? It makes more sense for us to take responsibility for finding out the facts, in a clear and methodical way, and to become meaningfully involved.

Consumers have inspired more humane and home-like birthing rooms in many hospitals. In these units, soft music and lighting, along with more comfortable beds, have replaced the stirrups and fluorescent lights.

We all have a backlog of 'medical material'. This refers to our unresolved emotions related to previous medical experiences. I can recall one painful memory of being in the hospital as a teenager, with my leg in a full cast, hanging by a pulley system on my bed, when a group of interns came on 'grand rounds' to examine my situation. Well, it wasn't so grand for me! Without any warning, they threw back the bedcovers and exposed my body, including the bloody menstrual pad I had not had time to rearrange. I felt like a piece of meat hanging in a marketplace.

All of our patients have had humiliating and painful experi-

228

ences related to their medical treatment in the past. Most of us, as nurses, also carry these memories, and we often have related symptoms in our bodies. For me, it has been in my throat and neck. For you, it may be stomach or head. Maybe you have a tennis elbow that won't heal, or intermittent burning in your stomach, but most people have their own personal warning signals that something is going on internally for them. As nurses, we can inspire healing in our patients and ourselves by paying attention to our emotional and physical symptoms.

Remember that we have said healing happens from the inside out. If we are conspiring to heal the medical system, it will happen from inside out as well as from the outside in. This is not a time to point fingers, but rather a time for action.

3. Change your mind and change the world.
Replace those painful or victimizing images with more healthy images. If you need to yell and scream and throw things to get beyond anger, do it in a safe and nurturing environment. Do not underestimate the power of healing with a well-trained psychotherapist who has worked on herself and is not afraid or confused by your strong emotions. From time to time, most people find themselves in need of guidance, emotional release, and mentorship from someone who has travelled a similar road.

As a psychiatric nurse and therapist, I have found it extremely useful to periodically enlist the support of a counselor or mentor, often in times of crisis. I have always been a very emotional person, and was made to believe that my emotionality was a shortcoming in me, a handicap. I have now come to see it as a great strength. My emotional

229

life has not changed; what has changed is the way I perceive this quality in myself, and my willingness to face squarely my own shortcomings and gifts.

I encourage you to begin to view your qualities as strengths, no matter what you have been told about yourself. Our negative images of ourselves have usually come from someone else's judgements about us, and should not be misconstrued as how we feel about ourselves. Each person is entitled to their own opinion about us, but ultimately we do not need to change unless we make the decision to do so for our own health and welfare.

Consider that the very qualities that you have been told are weaknesses may be judged so only by people who have been upset by your style. Perhaps they have been upset because they resent your freedom to be yourself. When people have given up their true selves, and tried to conform to societal expectations, they often carry a sense of loss and resentment. Do not allow their sense of impotence to color your views of yourself.

For exactly this reason, it is crucial that every person learn to take quiet inward time to reflect upon her/his own life, and evaluate how she/he feels about it, rather than become confused with the external messages. The internal ones, that wise healer inside you, seek full expression in order that you may make your greatest contributions to the conspiracy.

Remember, a conspiracy such as this is made of many unique and powerful individuals, each of whom makes a very special and important contribution to the whole. Do not be discouraged from being your own self, for that in itself is an act of courage, and also allows for the greatest possible healing for the greatest number of people.

How A Sensible Person Might Begin to Use These Diverse Suggestions

In healing, no one single maneuver will serve each patient as well as the combination of several approaches in a tailor-made program. Many people, for instance, neglect the mental and spiritual dimensions by erroneously concluding that nutrition and/or exercise alone is the true path. Others may focus on spirituality only, woefully neglecting growth on the other dimensions. Each is important; none alone is sufficient.

Remember to be at ease with however long the process of restoring health seems to take. Cures of a lasting nature, like any enduring change, take place in their own time and at their own speed. Many people, for example, are in such a hurry to lose weight quickly that they spend years and years losing and regaining, losing and regaining. This same yo-yo effect occurs with smoking, exercise, and countless other health activities. To get beyond this frustrating rhythm, make your changes gradually. Remember, too, the saying 'A journey of a thousand miles begins with a single step.'

Growing is a health process; Health is a growth process. May you find the wind always at your back on this magnificent journey into healing.

Summary

Just as Florence Nightingale worked to eliminate the source of physical disease, so can today's nurse, with consumer support, work to eliminate the mental anguish that plagues our culture. Just as she and a small team of nurses dragged a decaying dead horse out of the hospital water supply, so too could today's nurses (with consumer help) eliminate the 'decaying horse' of inappropriate technology and spiritual apathy.

With one foot in the door, yet not attached to the present medical system, today's nurses can lead the health care consumers through some powerful and necessary changes. Now is the time for nurses and consumers to team up, and join forces for a healthier tomorrow.

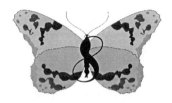

NURSE EMPOWERMENT
HEALING OURSELVES
AND OUR PROFESSION

"Nursing is an art, and if it is to be made an art, it requires as exclusive a devotion, as hard a preparation, as any painter's or sculptor's work; for what is the having to do with dead canvas or cold marble compared with having to do with the living body - the temple of God's spirit? It is one of the Fine Arts; I had almost said, the finest of the Fine Arts . . ." Florence Nightingale

We have explored the many problems in our present medical system. We have heard the stories of a nurse, doctor, and patient in their painful medical contacts. We have been witness to what has not worked.

Now, we are preparing to pave the way for a brighter future. We have learned from many of our mistakes, and are learning more every day about what constitutes true health. As nurses, we are in the

235

process of re-educating ourselves in order to soon take our proper place in the emerging paradigm.

To now discuss the emerging role of nursing in the 21st - century, we need to explore one of the key concepts in today's massive recovery movement, the issue known as 'codependency'. To become healthy role models for our patients, nurses must overcome dysfunctional patterns and move into more powerful behaviors.

Nurses Who Care Too Much

Earlier, in Chapter Two, I mentioned the recent proliferation of books and articles on 'codependency'. In an article in the *American Journal of Nursing*, Sara F. Hall, R. N., M.S.N., and Linda M. Wray R.N., M.S.N., describe the characteristics of the codependent nurse. Several identifying behaviors include the following:

1. Caretaking (meeting others' needs while neglecting her own)
2. Perfectionism (need to keep every aspect of her life under control; constant criticism of herself and others)
3. Denial (refusing to acknowledge painful parts of her life; ignores problems)
4. Poor communication (talks freely about others, holds back information about herself).[63]

According to the authors, these nurses are manipulative, blaming, and threatening, with inauthentic communication styles. They are overworked and over-committed. Because of unmet dependency needs, they tend to put on a strong front, further denying themselves what they might need to feel better.

Low self-esteem has inspired them to need to be needed, for they feel unworthy of life's blessings. To avoid thinking about their problems, they keep busy even in the face of mounting pressures, often engaging in workaholism or other addictions. As they dig deeper and deeper into these unhealthy patterns, they become more and more removed from their true feelings, living instead with a larger amount of denial about their pain.

Codependency can be considered the Achille's heel of the nursing profession. It is often described as an insidious disease, stemming from childhood wounding or neglect, that eats away at the strength and esteem of the individual, eroding the very fabric of their sense of well-being. As nurses, we need to become sharply aware of the ways in which our collective weaknesses have undermined our attempts at professionalization and collaboration, particularly if we are ultimately conspiring to empower health care consumers.

As an example, we can look at one of the many ways in which our damaged esteem as women impedes nursing's progress. When I make presentations to nursing groups, I often spark interest by exclaiming that if I were a physician, or administrator, or member of any group which might feel threatened by the empowerment of nurses, I would structure nursing education exactly the way it has been. As mentioned earlier, we have the one-year nurse, the two-year nurse, the three-year diploma nurse, the four-year baccalaureate nurse, the Clinical Nurse Specialist, the Nurse Practitioner, the Ph.D. Nurse Educator, etc.

Who wouldn't be confused? I don't know your experience, but I am a graduate of a four-year program, and was told that "we were the real nurses; the others aren't as good". This divisive approach has been extremely effective at preventing nurses from joining forces and conspiring for better care.

It also seems apparent that nurses (as a predominantly female group) have been greatly influenced by the masculine-oriented culture, learning very early from many subtle and overt experiences, that our value is less than that of males. These beliefs have served to foster jealously, envy, and competition among women, and nursing as a group is known for its 'catty' behavior. It is a rare nurse who escapes without being gossiped about, provoked, or demeaned by her fellow nurses. These incidents undermine our confidence, disempower us, and provide the temptation for us to retaliate, all of which are harmful to us.

~   ~   ~   ~   ~

I was 'relieved' of my position as a hemodialysis nurse many years ago, and the story warrants discussion at this juncture. I had just moved out to San Francisco, the land of my dreams, and was eager to begin my new life, after a divorce. Boldly, I applied for a technologically-challenging position, having become somewhat jaded by the crazy world of psychiatry. It was a happy day when I announced to my roommates that I had been accepted to work on a hemodialysis unit near one of the major medical centers in the country.

Things went well for the first month or two. I seemed to quickly acquire the skills to put the people on the machines, and to monitor them carefully. I found the job exciting and demanding, and was relieved to discover that all of my psychiatric training was needed to help support people with fatal kidney disease. I truly enjoyed having the opportunity to spend five hours, three times a week talking to them about their lives, and knew I was able to offer solace and wisdom. Also, the medical director seemed to truly respect my abilities.

238

Then, one day, Anne returned. I had heard about her, but had never had the pleasure of meeting her. Anne was the head nurse on the unit, and I was hired in her absence, as she had contracted hepatitis while working in dialysis. I found her to be amusing, sarcastic, and insecure. It didn't take her long to start finding things to complain about with my work. First it was indirect jokes, and soon her behavior was blatantly hostile. I tried on several occasions to discuss this with her, and her response was to deny anything other than the specific incident under discussion.

Finally, I was called into the medical office, where Dr. Grady informed me that there seemed to be a lot of disturbance about me on the unit. He admitted to being perplexed about it, as he and I had often worked side by side, and he had previously told me he had great respect for the way I worked with people. After a hefty sigh, he said, "I think it's Anne. She did not participate in hiring you, and feels threatened that you're young, attractive, and have a Master's degree. Frankly, I'm in a bind. She has said that either you go or she goes, and it's much more difficult to fill the head nurse position on this unit. I'm afraid I've had to make a business decision to let you go."

I was devastated. After spending most of my life achieving straight A's in school, I was fired from one of my first nursing positions because another nurse did not know how to handle her own insecurities. Granted, as Dr. Grady also said, I have a strong personality, and people either love me or hate me. I still felt a deep sense of wounding at not having the opportunity for Anne and I to work it out like two mature women.

Patriarchy has done little to stimulate growth among women. In fact, one of the more humorous aspects of this situation occurred when I finally came out of my shock and decided to apply for unemployment until I could find another job. The employment officer asked me why I was let go, and I could not seem to come up with a logical answer. She became exasperated, and called the dialysis unit where I had worked. After being put on hold four times, with a different voice answering each time, she demanded to know why I had been fired. She listened to the person talking on the receiver, then threw the phone into its cradle muttering something about 'crazy'. When I inquired as to what they had said, she looked at me and laughed. "They said you were 'unconsciously seductive'. What's the matter, honey, don't you like to sleep with the boss?" She quickly filled out the forms on her desk, and I was granted the gift of unemployment benefits.

A doctor once told me that he had a picture of both Florence Nightingale and William Osler hanging in his office. He noted that whenever a doctor came into the office, he usually spoke in admiration of the famous doctor. The nurses, on the other hand, almost invariably said "Did you know she died of syphilis?". He felt the nurses conveyed an attitude of disrespect and non-support for their own kind. It is certainly possible that doctors are trained to stick together and be supportive of each other, whereas nurses have learned to fight, and compete, and demean each other.

Another facet of the same problem is related to the escalating battle between nurse-midwives and lay midwives. Apparently many of the 'legitimate', certified nurse-midwives feel resentful and insecure about the lay midwives encroaching upon their territory. We have to examine this kind of behavior, however, and ask ourselves whether we are becoming part of the problem or part of the solution.

I can personally relate to this battle strongly, because I have often dreamed of becoming a certified nurse-midwife, yet I have not been able to find it in my heart to pursue a philosophy of birthing that has been generated by educated males. It somehow does not make sense to me! To me, birthing is sacred female work, and I believe that men should be invited in when they exhibit the qualities of wisdom, compassion, and deep reverence for the special powers of women to recreate life. Birth, after all, is a joyous rite of passage, a holy transition from one level of existence to another.[64] It is a spiritual journey, and needs to be honored as such.

For many centuries, women have cared for each other in giving birth, thus promoting the very female bonding we so desperately need in today's world. Birthing provides one more example of how women have given up what is undeniably our power to a masculine, authoritative system which has demeaned and devalued something holy.

In her book *On Nursing: Toward A New Endowment,* Margretta M. Styles, ex-Dean of The School of Nursing at UCSF, makes a distinction between 'professionhood' and 'professionalism'.[65] In her view, the first refers to the individual characteristics of any member of the profession, whereas the latter makes reference to the composite character of the profession. She feels strongly that for nursing to achieve professionalism, professionhood must precede it. In other words, as each nurse accepts responsibility for her individual contributions to the profession, we will then be empowered professionally as a group. As each nurse works toward her own self-actualization, she contributes to nursing's success.

It seems that in all professions, the women who make it to the top have had to fight long and hard not to be beaten down by a demoralizing system, and along the way have acquired some painful scars. Because of the nature of women's relationships with other women, we seem to save much of our repressed rage to vent on other women. Maybe we inherently trust other women more, and thus allow ourselves to ventilate our hostilities on each other, or perhaps it is because we disrespect each other enough that we dump our anger on other women, but it is time for us to collectively stop it!

~   ~   ~   ~   ~

Codependency in nursing has accounted for a great omission. Strong nursing leadership had definitely been the missing ingredient in a 'health care' system. Our failure as nurses to assert ourselves, individually and collectively, has led to untold sorrow and frustration. Our unwillingness to see our special contributions, and to insist on making them, have weakened our medical system, allowing it to spin out of control.

Are you a nurse who has cared too much? Has your caring been unbalanced, in that it is other-directed? Is it not time for nurses to start caring for and about themselves more, especially now that we recognize how important our role-modeling is to other nurses and consumers?

Statements are offered in many articles and books, including David Willard, R.N. and Candace Snow's *I'm Dying to Take Care of You*,[66] claiming that large percentages of health professionals come from dysfunctional families. Nursing seems to be no exception to this claim.

In Snow and Willard's book, the authors state that "codependence creates harmful consequences for better than 80% of the nursing profession". They further elaborate,

"Codependence emerges as a learned set of behaviors exhibited by children raised in dysfunctional families. It leads us to esteem ourselves by what we do, what

242

we look like, or what we have, rather than by who we are. As nurses, it invites us to give away our power as a spiritual body of women and men to the perceived abusiveness of an unwieldy medical bureaucracy; to addictions, eating disorders, unhappy primary relationships, burnout, and physical and mental illness."[67]

Of major impact is the effect on our nursing endeavors:

"Lastly, and most importantly, as the result of professional expectations and the issues we bring to the profession from our families, nurses often adopt a mask of being in control and perfect. When we do this, the essence of true healing - an accepting connection with the body, mind and spirit of a patient - is blocked."[68]

Another nurse-author, Caryn Summers, speaks clearly about many of these issues, having interviewed nurses from all settings. She explores their own dependency and addiction issues, and further describes her own painful process of recovery from drug addiction:

"The road to recovery is a self-healing process, not a quick fix, but a slow and arduous road that demands . . . rigorous honesty, admission to powerlessness, letting go of control, and allowing a power greater than the small ego self to facilitate in the journey back to health. Recovery is offered to each of us in three small words: "Healer, heal thyself."[69]

Caryn's inspiring book encourages us, as nurses, to follow the path with the heart; to journey to our truest self, and to allow our work to be guided by that deeper wisdom.

Similarly, the concept I am suggesting for a 'nursing conspiracy' was first put forth by Marilyn Ferguson in her powerful book *The Aquarian Conspiracy:*

> "It is a conspiracy without a political doctrine. Without a manifesto. With conspirators who seek power only to disperse it, and whose strategies are pragmatic, even scientific, but whose perspective sounds so mystical that they hesitate to discuss it. Activists asking different kinds of questions, challenging the establishment from within."[70]

In the section on holistic health (Chapter Six), we examined some of the assumptions of the old and new paradigms of medicine, as also outlined in Marilyn Ferguson's book. 'Conspire' can mean 'to breathe with, or together'. We can now begin together to incorporate the principles of natural healing into our daily lives as nurses, in order to become powerful models of healing for our patients.

Empowerment: The Key to a Healthy Future

In their book called *Empowerment: The Art of Creating Your Life As You Want It*, David Gershon & Gail Straub make some bold statements:

> "Most of us settle for far less in ourselves than we are capable of achieving. We fall victim to impoverished dreams, dreams that don't begin to do justice to the potential we hold. We need to learn how to dream, how to boldly and courageously reach for our highest visions

244

. . . to harness the passion of your heart with the power of your mind and create your fullest expression of being human . . . Knowing your deepest heart can mean avoiding years spent pursuing other people's dreams . . . to see and create a compelling vision of the life you truly desire . . . to overcome those parts of yourself that can sabotage your intentions.

"Our culture is primarily pathologically based. It focuses on what is wrong with a person . . . a view of life in which each of us learns merely how to cope and fit in rather than to excel and move out . . .

". . . learn how to transform limiting beliefs and behavior patterns . . . to overcome difficult life situations . . . moving from pathology to vision. It is shifting our basic attitude toward life from problem-solving to vision-creating. It requires us to let go of the deep problem-oriented programming of our culture and accept the belief that we can and will create the life we want."[71]

Empowerment Studies

To fully understand the necessary involvement of nursing in empowerment, we can examine research conducted at Stanford University by psychologist Albert Bandura. Over a period of years, Dr. Bandura and his colleagues have been investigating this phenomenon.[72] He has questioned what it is, how it occurs, how it can be measured in humans, how perception affects one's sense of power, and what long-term benefits can be derived from empowerment.

For nurses, I can think of no other single topic more timely or helpful. For years, we have strived for more power in varied ways. Many nurses carry a deep sense of victimization, as women and as nurses, due to the societal treatment they have received. Nursing is no stranger to a sense of victimization. Our early history captures many experiences of martyrdom (often religiously inspired).

Today we continually hear co-workers complain of having "our power taken away". Perhaps you are a nurse who has felt powerless and beaten in your work. Perhaps you, too, went into nursing with a sense of being called on a grand mission, and now find yourself feeling demeaned, devalued, and confused.

The root problem concerns an obvious need for nursing as a whole to define itself. Not only is society confused about our role, but internally nursing is engaged in an active search for meaning. In reality, power is the ability to influence change, and nurses could be vastly powerful change agents. What we have lost is a large measure of our sense of meaning, our 'reason to be'.

In his renowned explanation of 'existential analysis', one of Europe's leading psychiatrists, Victor Frankl has examined the intangible factors that inspire the will to live. A survivor of Nazi concentration camps, Dr Frankl lost all that was dear to him in the Holocaust. He spent years concerning himself with the question of what it is that allows people to 'keep on being', and to remain productive in the face of great losses.

In his book, *Man's Search for Meaning,*[73] Dr. Frankl explains that the human will to live is influenced most deeply by our ability to ascertain, each person for him/ herself, what it is that we live for. As a psychotherapist, he asked how one can awaken in another the feeling that he or she is "responsible to life, however grim his circumstances may be".[74] I believe it is this issue which concerns us as nurses both personally and professionally.

It is my distinct impression that when nurses recapture their individual sense of meaning and self-worth, we can join forces to create a powerful collective force for change. As we believe in ourselves and our mission more strongly, we can model empowerment and inspire health care consumers to awaken their 'will to live'. In my mind, it is this intangible, immeasureable, act that defines and gives nursing its purpose. Let us see from Dr. Bandura's studies how this can occur.

In his initial work, Dr. Bandura explored the sense of efficacy (ability to make changes) in women who had spider phobias.[75] He studied the role of perceived control in stress situations. By measuring epinephrine and norepinephrine levels, it has been shown that when one perceives oneself as unable to cope with potential threat, events are felt as stressful.

> "To the extent that people believe they can prevent, terminate, or lessen the severity of aversive events, they have little reason to be perturbed by them . . . people who judge themselves inefficacious in coping with environmental threats dwell on their vulnerabilities, and perceive many situations as fraught with danger . . ."[76]

In earlier research, Bandura found that "The more efficacious they perceive themselves to be . . . the weaker the stress reactions they experience while anticipating or performing the activities."[77] He proceeded to provide 'mastery modeling', with experimenters demonstrating and teaching about characteristics of spiders, educating the spider-phobic subjects as to how to handle spiders in any situation. At periodic intervals, subjects were re-tested with the self-efficacy scale.

The results indicated that as we strengthen our beliefs in our ability to cope, catecholamine reactivity is diminished in tasks that were previously intimidating. In other words, when people believe they can exhibit control, they perceive the experience as non-dangerous. Participant 'modeling' was consistently powerful in imparting a strong sense of coping efficacy. (In modeling, one is shown what to do, then trained how to do it).

Next, Dr. Bandura examined perceived self-efficacy in relationship to one's ability to handle stressful situations. He was demonstrating two things: first, how our beliefs about ourselves affect psychosocial functioning; and second, how mastery modeling experiences enable us to deal more effectively with previously stressful situations.

In more recent research, Dr. Bandura suggests:

". . . personal and social change rely extensively on methods of empowerment. These approaches achieve their effects by equipping people with the requisite knowledge, skills, and resilient self-beliefs of efficacy to alter aspects of their lives over which they can exercise some control."[78]

To further examine this phenomenon, he tested the hypotheses that perceived self-efficacy allows for empowerment in the face of physical threats. To do this, he provided a situation for women to gain mastery of physical skills needed to defend themselves successfully against sexual assaults. His findings demonstrated that "mastery modeling enhanced perceived efficacy, decreased perceived vulnerability to assault and reduced . . . negative thinking and anxiety . . . These changes were accompanied by increased freedom of action."[79]

In other words, after women were shown how to defend themselves, and practiced sufficiently under safe conditions, they judged themselves much less vulnerable to victimization. In addition, they were able to distinguish safe from risky conditions. They had less negative thinking and experienced less anxiety. The results of these changes included an expanded sense of freedom - they were able to make decisions about their lives based on what they did or did not want to, as opposed to making decisions based on fear. The women saw that a self-assured manner and firm response could reduce the likelihood of assault. Thus, they also felt more competent to judge the riskiness of situations. According to Bandura, "The results of this study thus indicate that empowering people . . . serves both to protect and liberate them."[80]

How This Research Benefits Us As Nurses

Why is this empowerment research so crucial to the transformation of nursing in America today? Why should we, as nurses, inspire others to feel more powerful? How can we feel that way ourselves?

As nurses, and as women in a predominantly masculine culture, we often feel victimized by the system in which we operate. We have, as a group, allowed our consciousness to be bombarded by negative images and beliefs. We are made to feel 'less than', inferior, weaker than our male counterparts. Even male nurses often admit to identifying more with the physicians, the 'stronger' models. Yet, isn't it true that nursing was created out of a need to provide the tender nurturing care that often can make the difference between a patient's will to live or not?

Certainly the curative aspects of modern medicine have offered many people the chance to live - to beat illness and to live healthy, productive lives. But for many others, the dis-ease process seems to eat away at their spirit, leaving them feeling beaten and broken in a body that failed them. For these patients, fixing the body is not enough. Their sense of worth and value as a human being is diminished, and we nurses have been witness to the dark despair of people who might have overcome the physical manifestation of their illness, only to succumb to the compromised sense of self that often accompanies disability.

In military terms, it is like 'winning the battle but losing the war'. In fact, military terminology is very appropriate when examining the shortcomings of our present medical system. Much of illness in our society is treated as if it were a battle. The organism is the enemy, the doctor is the conquering hero, and the battleground - the patient! In our clearer moments of thinking about this approach, how can we, as nurses, be devoted to winning the war if we, and the patients, lose dignity and self-respect in that process?

Thus, as the Secretary's Commission on Nursing found, it is now up to us, as nurses, to emerge as powerful leaders in health care. It is our challenge to articulate who we are to a confused public, and to command their support for the mutual goals we share.

Where To Start

Question: What is missing and most needed in medicine today?

Answer: YOU! You are a missing ingredient in the conspiracy.

Let us remember that Napoleon Hill said all success begins with an idea. If you support the concept of joining forces to heal our health care system, then you can see the wisdom of beginning to see yourself as a vital part of the solution. The truth is that each of us has a purpose and brings special gifts to the conspiracy.

As we overcome any old sense of victimization, as we recognize fully who we are and what the task is, and as we claim our proper place in society, the balance will be returned. We, as nurses, are entrusted with the care of the consumers on a whole-person level. We are not only here to care for the body, but also the soul and spirit.

Empowerment occurs when we feel more efficacious, and recognize that we can get ourselves out of any unsafe situation. It comes from knowing that we have the skills, tools, information, and support with which to make healthy changes. It comes as we each personally empower ourselves, then model empowerment so nurses can learn from each other how to be strong and effective as leaders.

Empowerment studies can help support our journey from victimization to strong leadership, from non-assertiveness to clear strong communication, from a lesser position to an equal place in health care. They help because we now know that our attitudes about ourselves and our work directly create the outcome. These studies challenge us, as nurses, to be fully ourselves, and to show how powerful we truly are.

As a final thought on empowerment, what is power? According to Webster's Dictionary, power is *the ability to influence change.* Now that we nurses realize the urgent need for a great many healthy changes in our medical system, it is imperative that we join forces to create synergy. It is now time to convert our 'sick care system' into a true health care system, both for our patients' benefit, and for ourselves.

Empowerment Methods

In speaking to nurses about actually accomplishing empowerment, I have devised some of my own ideas as to what it would really look like for nursing to empower itself. To support understanding of these visions, I consider some of the concepts presented by Napoleon Hill in his empowering and best-selling book, *Think and Grow Rich.*[81]

As a struggling college student, Mr. Hill made his way through school by interviewing successful men to ascertain the secrets of power and success. As good fortune would have it, his first interviewee was Andrew Carnegie. Napoleon chose to apprentice under the mentorship of Mr. Carnegie, and spent the next twenty years organizing the Science of Personal Achievement. He carefully noted what qualities enabled an individual to become successful in meeting his own predetermined goals. Among some of his most noteworthy ideas are the following:

> 1. "Thoughts are things, and powerful things at that, when they are mixed with definiteness of purpose persistence, and a burning desire for their translation into . . . material objects."[82]

2. "Faith is a state of mind which may be induced, or created, by affirmation or repeated instructions to the subconscious mind, through the principle of autosuggestion."[83]

3. "Knowledge is only potential power. It becomes power only when, and if, it is organized into definite plans of action and directed to a definite end."[84]

4. ". . . First you give life and action and guidance to ideas, then they take on power of their own and sweep aside all opposition."[85]

5. "Every plan you adopt . . . should be the joint creation of yourself and every other member of your 'Master Mind' group . . ."[86]

6. "The 'Master Mind' may be defined as *Coordination of knowledge and effort, in a spirit of harmony, between two or more people, for the attainment of a definite purpose.*"[87]

7. "If the first plan which you adopt does not work successfully, replace it with a new plan . . . temporary defeat is not permanent failure . . . A quitter never wins - and a winner never quits."[88]

8. 'Power' may be defined as 'organized and intelligently directed knowledge'.[89]

He also stated some of the *major attributes of leadership*:

1. Unwavering courage based upon knowledge of self, and of one's occupation.

2. Self-control

3. A keen sense of justice

4. Definiteness of decision

5. Definiteness of plans (successful leader must plan his work, and work his plan)

6. The habit of doing more than paid for

7. A pleasing personality . . . leadership calls for respect

8. Sympathy and understanding

9. Mastery of detail

10. Willingness to assume full responsibility

11. Cooperation (must understand and apply the principle of cooperative effort. Leadership calls for power, and power calls for cooperation.)[90]

Hill then provides the following example of what can be accomplished when leadership and power combine:

"When a group of individual brains are coordinated and function in harmony, the increased energy created through that alliance becomes available to every

individual brain in the group . . . Mahatma Gandhi . . .
came by power through inducing over two hundred million people to coordinate, with mind and body, in a spirit
of harmony for a definite purpose . . . Gandhi accomplished a miracle . . . "[91]

~   ~   ~   ~   ~

Nurses often seem perplexed when I speak about Napoleon
Hill's concepts of 'Personal Achievement' during nursing seminars.
There seems to be a sense that nurses should not be involved in the
world of business and leadership. This 'sense' is 'non-sense', and
has contributed greatly to our lack of empowerment.

Nurses must understand that *we are in business*, the business of
providing health care to consumers. We may prefer to be like os-
triches, with our heads in the sand, but the fact remains that for
nursing to achieve empowerment, we must begin to collectively
focus on a more businesslike orientation.

There are newly-emerging organizations designed specifically
to inspire nurses to develop more collaboration. The National Nurses
in Business Association[92] has been a blessing for me and other nurse
entrepreneurs as we seek to empower ourselves as business people in
nursing. With national conferences twice annually, it provides a
forum for nurses to network and share knowledge and experience.

And of course, another major healing force in my professional
life has been the American Holistic Nurses Association.[93] To me,
this group epitomizes the 'Master Mind' that Mr. Hill so clearly
describes as a necessary ingredient for success. For many nurses, the
AHNA represents the heart-centered, nurturing group that we always
knew nurses could be, were we not isolated in stressful institutional

settings. We laugh, we cry, we sing and dance and hug and learn with each other at conferences several times a year. This nourishment sustains so many of us in our individual and group endeavors. Most important, the AHNA rekindles my belief that nursing is spiritual work.

Nurses in Transition, American Holistic Nurses Association, National Nurses in Business - each of these groups has become a source of strength and community for thousands of nurses seeking empowerment, knowledge, and spiritual connection. Is it not time we treat each other at least as well as we treat our patients? Having a place to go for skills, tools, information, and support has made all the difference to me as a nurse.

A Personal Story

I am no longer one isolated person in a megalithic institution - I am a unique person, honored and respected for the specific gifts and talents I bring to nursing. I feel like part of a sacred sisterhood, living in modern times, yet cherishing some of nursing's deepest held tenets regarding human life and death. I feel like a part of a grand social movement, destined to create major changes in our society. I am an important thread in the emerging tapestry of health care; I am a conspirator, and a change agent.

Once, when I was in graduate school, my highly theatrical nursing instructor stood up in front of the class and flapped her arms wildly. She repeatedly insisted that we try to understand our mission as 'change agents'.

"You all know about secret agents, right? Well, to be a change agent within the medical system is like being a special kind of secret agent."

She was right about that. It was such a secret that none of us knew what she was talking about! It was several years later, when I was working in hospitals that I began to grasp the concept. At the time, I was at a psychiatric facility which was part of a megacorporation. My assigned unit was a day treatment center, and I was hired as a nurse to help run the program.

It was awkward from the beginning, because the nurse who was my superior (once again) had not been consulted in the least as far as my hiring was concerned. As if that was not enough of a challenge, you should have seen her face when she read my nametag, ending in 'R.N., M.S.' Her name was Laura, and from the first day, she was out for blood - mine!

Laura was an R.N. from the 'old school', having been trained in a three-year diploma program. I, on the other hand, had just completed four years at a university and another two to acquire my Master's degree. As I said, I was in trouble from the moment I set foot in her doorway.

The strange thing was, I liked her. I wanted to be her friend, even though she was my boss. She made it apparent, however, that a friendly relationship was just not in the cards. She was sneaky, though, old Laura.

It has been said that nurses as a group have been passive-aggressive, having often viewed ourselves as victims. Victims tend to express their hostility and aggression covertly. So, one day early on, Laura came bounding into the room, announcing that she had a treat for me. Now, I've always loved treats.

257

"You know, I've been thinking," she began. "You mentioned when you first came that you really were eager to gain more first-hand experience leading therapy groups. Well, I have a surprise for you! As you may have heard, for several years I have had the distinct privilege of co-leading an evening group with one of the five directors of the Institute's corporation."

"His name is Dr. Tirent, and he's one of the chief psychiatrists in the company." I couldn't imagine where this build-up was about to lead. She continued, "Well, recently my husband asked me to join a skiing club which meets weekly to do projects, and those meetings happen to fall on the same night that we co-lead our group. I knew you'd be delighted, so I have taken the liberty of asking Dr. Tirent if he would interview you to ascertain whether you could replace me as the female leader. He so graciously offered you his 2:00 slot today."

She stopped, leaving me there with my mouth hanging open. What was I in for? I was terribly nervous; I never expected to be applying for co-leadership with one of the big honchos. I was not sure I was ready for that. As it turned out, however, he was not ready for me either!

As I knocked on the big wood door that bore the sign 'Cecil B. Tirent, M.D.', my knees knocked against each other under my dress. I walked in and was looked at (not greeted) by a man who seemed strangely like a hybrid between a billiard ball and a vacuum cleaner. Now, I realize that is an odd description, but he was round and bald, and he seemed to be taking in everything. (Maybe he was actually more like a tape recorder than a vacuum). The point is, he stared and stared at me, and offered minimal response. Now I saw how those analytical psychiatrists came to be called 'shrinks'. I nestled into a chair, hoping I would soon shrink away to nothingness. He seemed

258

to be scrutinizing everything about me, while somehow maintaining a far-away look.

The interview went as well as could be expected. At the end, after I had done all the talking, he stood up. It turns out he was a short fellow after all - perhaps with a Napoleon complex? I was amazed to see that my counter-defense was to scrutinize him! I was dismissed with a curt gesture, and he seemed to mumble something like "you'll do".

It gave me a distinctly creepy, yet vaguely familiar feeling. I soon identified it as a deep pervasive frustration, something I remember sensing in my mother during my younger years. I had the distinct feeling that I would come out of those groups feeling the way my mother must often have felt back then.

Though deeply loving, she was also an intense and extremely emotional person, who had married my father to balance out that side of herself. My father, not unlike many men of his era, was given to deep periods of pensive non-communication, much to her dismay. The combination was lethal . . .

So it was with that cheery beginning that I walked into my first group, Karilee Halo, R.N., Co-leader. One by one, people paraded into the room, each pulling up a chair which seemed to be preordained for that person. There was a great hush as all eyes fell on me.

Dr. Tirent sat down brusquely, scrutinized his fingernails on each hand from left to right, and began to chew on the one which beckoned him the most. After what seemed like a very long silence, someone made a profound statement. 'She's new'.

I introduced myself, and began to tell something about what I was here for, when with the slightest flick of his wrist he told me to stop. I stopped talking, and again a great silence fell upon the group. Eventually someone came up with something dismal to share, and the group proceeded with what seemed to be a comfortable format for them - comfortable in the sense of a well-worn shoe. I realized that this is how the group normally functioned, and I found myself yawning most of the way through. I felt very clear that Dr. Tirent wanted me to be quiet, yet I couldn't help but wonder why I was there.

I decided to ask him after the group meeting. Normally, after a therapy group, it is customary for co-leaders to remain and process together. For that reason, I was amazed to see Dr. T. walk out immediately at the stroke of nine. I ran after him.

"Dr. Tirent", I ventured, "may I have a moment with you?" (Aren't nurses amazingly polite?). He turned, stopped suddenly in his tracks, and looked at me.

"Yes?" Now we were getting somewhere, I thought. This was the most he had spoken to me yet. "Do you have a minute to post-group with me?"

"What for?" I began to come unglued. (Yep; this must surely have been how Mom felt.)

"I have some questions for you. I'm not sure how you would like for me to react."

"Your job is not to react. Just sit there. We just need a female body." (Could I believe my ears?)

"I don't understand," I said. "Surely I have more to offer than that."

"Don't waste your breath. It's not necessary. You don't have to understand. Just be there, that's all. If you can't do that, don't be

260

there. It's simple."

I was infuriated. I hadn't gone through six years of college and all that nursing just to sit there like a bump on a log. Who died and made him boss, anyhow?

I swallowed my retort, turned away, and got myself out of there. The cool night air awakened my sensibilities. Perhaps he too needed some healing and understanding. I decided that I would try to play by his rules for a while.

Nonetheless, after some time I still concluded that his group was one of the least therapeutic I had ever seen. Week after week, I tried to be a female body in the co-leader's chair, and week after week, I grew to wonder more and more how this diminutive person had been granted such power. He rarely spoke, and when he did, he would come across in a highly superficial manner. He would give answers to meaningful questions by saying something like "It's because of your paranoid nature." To me, he was living proof of the Peter Principle in action; he had been promoted to his proper level of incompetence.

Finally, summer approached, and the last meeting of this group was held. They would take the summer off, then consider whether to 're-up' or not. It was a time for ending, and I decided that my final gift would be to share my thoughts and feeling from the heart just this once.

I started talking, and before I knew it, my mouth went on automatic pilot, as the words struggled to make their escape at long last. I must have talked for a very long time, for finally I heard a sharp, loud "SHUT UP!" It startled me, and my barrage stopped instantly. I looked around, and saw eight pairs of lit-up, thoughtful eyes where only marbles had been before. For the first time, I was truly making contact with all the other 'bodies' in that room - all but one. I felt warm and flushed, and a quick look at Dr. T. told me I could also feel finished.

Some good did come out of it, however. First, this time it was the good doctor himself asking for (demanding) a post-group session. We sat in his office, and he proceeded to lecture me about my horrendous behavior. I barely heard the lecture, but I was able to hear these words which followed:

"You told me when you first came that you were taught in your graduate program to be a change agent. I must say that I don't approve of your methods, but you have been successful. You've definitely changed things since you came here. People are agitated. I'm not sure it will ever be the same!"

Well, I suspect that was not intended to be a compliment, but I decided to accept it as one anyhow. To me, the patients and staff appeared more animated, not agitated. Perhaps that is splitting hairs, but I was glad to have been there, and felt that if things were more humane after I left, then I had been successful.

In looking back, it is easier to see how frightened and insecure he was. I can also imagine the extreme stresses on psychiatrists, and why they might choose 'professional detachment' in their relationships. I truly hope he has since achieved a deeper acceptance of himself and a more humane approach to his work. Peace to you, Dr. T.

~   ~   ~   ~   ~

I see a great need for nurses and doctors today to create places to work on their feelings about each other separately and together. Each of us has learned and developed attitudes about the role of the other, attitudes in need of healing. If we are to inspire patients to be their fullest selves in every sense of the word, then we must strive for that goal, modeling health accurately ourselves.

Part of my dream is to have the opportunity to travel with my physician-husband, using emotional release experiences in institutional settings, so doctors and nurses can heal their 'medical material'. As we do this together, we will also learn how to allow these healing releases in our patients, many of whom come to us with a multitude of fears and mistrusts based on their previous experience.

In making ourselves more real and vulnerable together, we will also be inspiring a new model of collaboration. The male/female, doctor/nurse polarities can be safely explored and transformed, freeing us all from the bondage of unrealistic, unhealthy expectations and roles. Learning, as health professionals, to release our emotional charge will offer us infinite possibilities for wellness - as individuals, as professionals, and as healers.

Are nurses ready to release our fears and mistrusts surrounding doctors? This is the place for us to begin. How about support groups? Would you like to get together with other nurses and begin to see each other as real people, with real problems, and real solutions? You can even begin by asking a nurse to join you for tea. Many on-going support groups have had very humble beginnings, and eventually shaped themselves into an ongoing experience, often with a regular 'core' group, and plenty of options for people to be involved regularly or to come and go as they wish. The AHNA has state coordinators and local networks, and guidelines for starting support groups. Take your step in your own way.

Removing Our Masks

I can also recall my nursing instructors trying to teach us to develop that professional detachment early in our program. I distinctly remember having the feeling that in order to be a good nurse, I was to put on a mask for the beginning of each shift, and peel it off when I was done, maybe in the comfort of my own home. The 'mask of professionalism' was always an enigma to me. I just didn't seem to know how to put it on and take it off perfectly at will, and could not even understand why they wanted us to do it that way.

I knew that nursing required sensitivity and compassion, and felt that I offered some of my greatest strengths in sharing these. Why would they want me to cover up my true self, and hide who I really am? Was I unacceptable the way I was? Was something wrong with the 'real me'?

Today, I have learned methods to protect myself and insure my safety amidst psychic bombardment, and I often have to use this skill with co-workers as much as patients. My goal is to have my personal life and my nursing life coexist as smoothly and peacefully as possible. I do not want to hide behind a mask, and try to fool everyone into thinking I'm anything other than a real person, with real feelings, trying to do a real and meaningful job. (Anyone else out there feel that way?)

I now realize that the role of a change agent is not an easy one. In my early life, as one of five children, I learned that 'the squeaky wheel gets the grease'. In my family, we each adopted roles, and I was the outspoken one, sharer of feelings and truth. I was destined to be a 'master change agent'.

Now that I've learned more about the nature of change, however, I realize that a designated change agent is only the spark, the idea-person, the mouthpiece. My work cannot succeed alone. I must also entice others around me to speak their truths, to share their feelings and guidance.

Now, I am reaching out to the nurses of America. Does anyone out there have strong feelings about the way things have been? Does anyone have any ideas about promoting healthy changes? Let's imagine that we have all joined forces, and are conspiring to create a more healing environment in the world of medicine. Where might we choose to start? To me it's obvious . . .

Changing our Image: How to Start

First, we must learn to empower and care for ourselves. We need to awaken our own healing potential, to feel better more of the time, and to begin to provide healthy models of empowerment. Then, and only then, can we inspire the consumers of American health care to join in the conspiracy.

I have discussed the importance and methods of consumer empowerment. We nurses cannot help inspire a consumer awakening until we join forces as powerful healthy role-models. We must change our image.

Today, many nursing organizations are receiving large donations to promote the image of nursing, and have provided television spot announcements and other media presentations. The National League of Nursing conducted a writing campaign in recent years to the sponsors of a television show which downgraded the image of the caring nurse into a brainless sexpot. As a result, several sponsors abandoned the project and the show was cancelled, providing a small example of what can happen when we speak out.

On the national level, individual states are organizing committees to consider proposals for change. Hospitals are madly advertising for nurses, each claiming to be caring environments for the nurses. Hospitals are likewise experimenting with improved nursing flexibility.

How can the individual nurse become involved?

The paths are many. Begin by speaking out in whatever situation you find yourself, Speak publicly when possible. Write to the media, offering or withdrawing support for their projects as you deem it necessary. More nurses are obviously needed as media consultants, so if you have always wanted to be involved in drama or theater, this may be your chance!

Constantly be aware of what you are saying about nursing through thought, word, and deed. Strive to project the aspects of nursing which demonstrate teamwork, teaching ability, integrity, authority, clear communications, and personal power.

Remember to support and reach out to nurses who are helping to enhance a powerful image, while likewise being outspoken when we're portrayed poorly. Mutual support is *crucial* in this massive undertaking. You may be inspired to start your own peer support group. If so, constantly strive to guide participants toward positive change. Also, steer clear of prolonged gripe sessions or individual counseling in the group setting.

Contribute wherever you find yourself. Write editorials and letters to people in influential positions. Convince your friends to boycott movies or television shows which demean your profession. We can only be guardians of the public welfare if we are willing to guard our own honor and integrity. Let us each do our best to remain clear and compassionate as we move towards a more balanced health care system.

NOW IS THE TIME TO STOP FIGHTING OURSELVES. NOW IS THE TIME TO SETTLE OUR INTERNAL STRIFE. NOW IS THE TIME TO HEAL THE BLEEDING IN OUR SOULS, TO RETURN TO THE SOURCE OF OUR POWER.

Surely we can diminish the possibility of extinction by finding those threads which unite us in our work. We must locate them, no matter how fine they are, and strengthen them, weaving a web of protection and clarity around us as we forge into our future. The decision remains with you - and with each and every nurse.

Aren't we finally tired of backbiting? Haven't we grown in our ability to recognize the many ways in which that is devouring our dreams? Now we can remember how important it is to listen to our hearts, to ease the conflict created when the outer demands do not agree with the still small voice inside. Now we can move forward together, one step at a time, one day at a time, each nurse at her own pace.

Now we can begin to appreciate our special strengths, our commitment, and our courage. It is especially time to honor our feminine aspects (male and female nurses) - those long-forgotten, undernourished parts of ourselves which cry out in hunger. We need food for our souls, that we may remember how to provide that for others.

Jumping Right In

The challenge starts here - it begins today - and it starts with you. Too long have we squabbled over the entry level for nursing. Too long has lack of convenient matriculation within our ranks been allowed to undermine our cohesion. We must provide ways for nurses to receive inspiration and incentives at all points on their journey.

In this vast undertaking, let us enlist the support of our government, and the media, and any other group in a position to benefit from our efforts. This includes many, for our society as a whole stands to gain in great measure from a cohesive nursing force, and we must inspire each faction in its own way.

We now exist in a time when technological advances and funding dictate policy in caring. We are managers of health care, providing essential services to humans in crisis. As hospitals continue to expand and take over entire city blocks, and the amount spent on one single piece of machinery would pay more than 100 nurses' salaries for a full year, we have continued to live in our time-warp, oblivious to our own naivete.

Hospital corporations are providing some of us with management training, which can be extremely valuable. However, some nurses report that they're receiving training often with subliminal

268

messages that they are to help keep the other nurses from speaking out. How much longer will we close our eyes to the realities, allowing ourselves to be the hospital maid-service thrown in with room and board? Again, it is no one's fault, merely the way of massive institutionalization.

I remember my organizational sociology professor standing in front of us, pointing to a huge organizational chart on the wall. "Tell me which box you select on this chart, and I will tell you the characteristics of that person." No room for individuality in these major systems.

I know these are strong pronouncements, but I want to get my point across. I am a nurse, and proud to be a nurse, and feel strongly that we can only improve our image and conditions by working together. I, too, have attended management training programs, and been wined and dined to keep my staff compliant. But there came a time when I could no longer ignore the knot in my throat and I could no longer contain my rage.

Since that time, I have done a lot of healing on myself. I have worked through much of the anger, and am now able to transform that intense emotional energy into action. I have met hundreds, perhaps thousands of nurses like myself, and I know there are hundreds of thousands of you out there who know exactly what I'm talking about. Do you want to continue to feel overworked and overwhelmed, undernourished and underappreciated, because we cannot decide whether we are professionals or not?

All people in leadership positions find that in order to be successful, they must take risks, be responsible, and convey power. In being painfully honest, don't we feel, deep in our heart of hearts, somewhat responsible for the anguish of health care consumers who have been overpowered by technological abuse? This submerged guilt could account for much of our self-flagellation, disrespect, and allowing ourselves not to have what we deserve.

In some ways, we have neglected to protect the public's welfare through our disease of codependency, and our fear of speaking out. Aren't we truly the patients' advocate, the one left to decipher 'medical-ese' and translate it into something meaningful for our clients? Isn't it actually a part of our work to balance out medical care?

Yes, medicine has been changing in the last century, with technology as the driving force, and big money as the stakes. The consumers are paying the price. But we nurses know the stakes have been much, much higher, to nurses and doctors as well as consumers. We've seen lives lost through greed, lives botched through ignorance and lack of accountability, and a diminished quality of life for many people facing the most challenging human transitions, especially birth and death.

Where has nursing been throughout these excesses? We have unwittingly become accomplices, watching the lure of money and power usurp the most valuable human experiences and turn them into profit for the medical-industrial complex (not even for ourselves!).

We do not need to further blame or criticize ourselves, though there are times we must face the realities squarely in order to heal. What is important now is to do something about it. Our codependency role as silent partners in the medical monopoly has arisen as a natural consequence of abdicating our power, and thus no longer being heard. (There is even a nursing group named after the wise soothsayer, Cassandra, who always gave accurate prophecies, but was never believed. Also, as mentioned earlier, Florence Nightingale wrote a little-known, yet *profound* essay: "Cassandra: Angry Outcry Against the Forced Idleness of Victorian Women").

We now need to be more positive and trusting. Know that if enough of us speak out the truth, we will be listened to and heard. The time has also come to be more active. If you have never belonged to a professional group, try it. If you do not feel positive about what they are doing, inspire them to stretch and change. Remain focused on the goals of *nursing's powerful image and nurse support.*

In your own way, become vocal, and do your part to help nursing reclaim its collective voice. Every nurse can have major impact on a failing system, so motivate others to assist in nursing's transformation.

Begin with *your* single step - whatever it is - and start today to build a healthier tomorrow.

Reaching Our Fullest Potential

As we gather tools to insure success in our healing endeavors, we must come to understand some of the aspects of power. Power can be defined as *an ability to compel obedience, to wield coercive forces, control or dominion over something.* Likewise, it can be seen as *energy, strength, or might; that which possesses substantial influence.* To empower, therefore, is *to give official authority to something; to enable.*

Self-empowerment is giving power to ourselves. It is a conscious process of reminding ourselves of that which we already

271

possess. Through the empowerment process, we enable ourselves to feel our power. It has always been there; no one can take it away. What we have given away, however, has been our innate ability to be and feel powerful. In this light, the process of empowerment is something that should come naturally to us as nurses. We have been reminding others of their power to heal themselves, and have forgotten (oops!) to heal ourselves!

Recent research in self-healing demonstrates that when people believe they really do have control over what happens in their lives, they have less pain associated with their illness. Those who feel powerless, even though performing exercises and learning information, often do not truly benefit from their therapies. As we have seen, it has been documented that the release of the body's chemical messengers is influenced by a person's sense of empowerment.

Medical doctors involved in holistic health modalities have been studying the process and using the information as they care for patients. Dr. Tom Ferguson, editor of *Medical Self-Care* magazine, feels that empowerment is the key to healing, and that the caregiver must offer tools, skills, information, and support for self-help. Dean Ornish, M.D., President of San Francisco's Preventive Medicine Institute, believes that feelings of isolation and loneliness contribute to stress-related disease, while increasing one's intimate connections can lead to empowerment. Nursing is greatly appreciative of physicians who carry these beliefs!

Now is the time for nurses to increase our sense of control and effectiveness in the world. We can begin this process in almost any arena of our daily lives. We can start empowering ourselves by seeing nurses as strong, powerful and whole. We can begin to notice our thoughts, now that we understand how our thoughts contribute to realities, and we can consciously go about the work of changing our thought habits to serve our needs. We can certainly change our 'self-talk', the messages we give ourselves through inner dialogue.

Since we are creatures of habit, one of the empowering concepts being taught on all levels of business is that we can replace our harmful habits with empowering ones. Our brain, like a computer, stores endless information, and can be programed with positive thoughts, the old ones deleted as they no longer serve. We can, for example, replace our downtrodden thoughts with more upbeat ones.

In Steven Covey's book Principle Centered Leadership[94] he says: "If we learn to manage things and lead people, we will have the best bottom line, because we will unleash the energy and talent of people . . . We will inspire others through advancing ourselves . . . "[95]

He also defines the Eight Characteristics of Principle Centered Leaders:

> "Continually learning, service oriented, radiate positive energy, believe in other people, lead balanced lives, see life as an adventure, synergistic, and they exercise for self-renewal".[96]

When you reflect on your work as a nurse, if you feel content, you are likely to convey that to others. Let people know by your healthy attitude, your proud posture, and your clear work choices that you are happy to be a nurse. Treat yourself and others with a respect born of professionalism and a valued sense of esteem. The nursing community will feel proud to associate with you, for you remind us all of our rich heritage.

Then you will be helping to portray an image of nursing that is competent and confident. That alone will go a long way towards helping to inspire others to join us in nursing. With each part contributing to the whole picture, it is essential that you recognize how *very, very* important you are in the transformation of nursing. Every single nurse counts; every nurse makes a difference. It is a ripple effect . . .

Follow Your Heart: New Avenues to Pursue

If you want to take another big step towards healing nursing's image, imagine yourself doing what your heart tells you is the perfect nursing job for you - your heart's desire. Take time to imagine it, to dream it up, to fantasize and play with ideas. Maybe you can see yourself doing massages and sharing herbal information with people on luxury cruise ships. That does not have to remain just a dream. To you it may be, but there are nurses doing that work now.

Maybe you want to run a summer camp for disabled children. I know of a few nurses who have worked to create that for themselves. Many nurses are pursuing advanced degrees and certifications in the various related healing arts, such as chiropractic, deep tissue work, imagery.

I am presently enrolled in two certification programs, both offered through the AHNA, that are very exciting to me. One will allow for me and thousands of other nurses to demonstrate competency and become Certified Healing Touch Practitioners, the other as Certified Holistic Nurses. Each of these programs meets in weekend or week-long gatherings at intervals to allow for the integration and practice of new tools learned.

Once you pursue either advanced degrees or certifications, you can add those skills to your nursing practice. Some nurses are in

274

private practice, taking these newly-acquired skills to help people heal in their communities and homes.

Empowerment means telling the truth. We have always known that nursing is so very much more than being hand-maidens to doctors. With our large, compassionate hearts, we have managed to take on many of medicine's problems, often unconsciously. There has never been a time when it's been more crucial, or more possible, to clearly define nursing. We have suffered greatly for forgetting who we are.

I must repeat: *Nursing is an art, separate from medicine.* Nursing licensure grants nurses power to deal with issues of health. It is infinitely more than caring for people in hospitals. In fact, Florence Nightingale said that hospitals were never intended to take in the whole sick population, rather, that they are an intermediary step.

In their landmark book *Nurse Abuse*, editors Laura Gasparis and Joan Swirsky offer many possible nursing solutions, covering academic, political, feminist, business, marketing, legal, and psychological arenas. They conclude:

> "The current crisis in nursing - indeed the future
> of nursing - can be resolved if we invoke the philosophy
> of 'Nurse-Heal thyself'. It is time to turn our full atten-
> tion, not to the image we have had, but to the substance
> that we have. Nursing must take a hard and critical look
> at itself, acknowledge its flaws, and then embark on
> revolutionary measures of change."[97]

Nursing must be involved with promoting the patient's sense of well-being, in assisting and supporting them in strengthening their own constitution to ward off disease. Where we work is vitally important, so it is time to put more attention to the health aspects of our work environments.

Nurses are in a perfect position to become prevention experts. We can capitalize on the public's recent interest in staying healthy, and make ourselves useful to corporations who would like to offer better health benefits to employees. This is actually smart business, cost effective because we can help people feel better, work better, and enjoy it more.

If you feel inspired to learn more about prevention, and to teach these concepts to the public, you may become a health promoter and educator. In working towards that goal, start seeking out continuing education classes which teach holistic principles and practice. If you have already learned a lot about this, start teaching classes to inspire other nurses to learn more about natural alternatives. Even if you continue to work within the medical model, you will be in a better position to assist patients and doctors should they decide to experiment with less toxic therapies.

Remember, even if you've never studied these concepts in nursing school, you have a broad base of health orientation from which to operate and grow. The process of seeking out this information is very empowering, and has its own built-in reward system, in that you learn more about yourself and feel better. Nurses can begin on any level, and ultimately arrive at a position of health mastery. If you work in a hospital setting, such as in medical-surgical or rehabilitation, be sure to speak out to make sure the nurses you work with are as respected and well-treated as nurses in the more 'prestigious areas' (critical care, telemetry, etc.).

Have you been curious about the role of the mind in healing?

Never has there been a more suitable time to study this topic. In recent years there has been an explosion of books and tapes on visualization, self-hypnosis, mindpower, and mental imagery. Many doctors who have begun to incorporate this into their practice are seeing the benefits of these as powerful adjuncts to medical treatment, and also as healing tools in their own right.

These methods inspire the body to muster its forces towards health. Using these tools at the bedside, patients feel more relaxed and powerful over their pain, decreasing the need for possibly harmful medicines. Many nurses are using relaxation techniques at the bedside to eliminate the need for sleep medications, and find that it is a relaxing job benefit for themselves as well!

Many nurses today are also returning to the ancient custom of gathering knowledge of nature's remedies, particularly herbs and foods, to strengthen and support healing. Nurses are also learning and using Therapeutic Touch as taught through certification programs nationwide, and in graduate level nursing classes at New York University, initiated by Dr. Delores Krieger. Therapeutic Touch, and Healing Touch (as taught in programs offered through the American Holistic Nurses Association), work with the energy field surrounding the body, promoting enhanced energy available to the client.

Many of these traditions come from other times, and other places. We, in the United States, are truly a young nation when comparing ourselves to cultures steeped in more ancient wisdom. We have much to learn from China, Japan, India, and other parts of the world, for they offer thousands of years of history in their healing techniques.

Like the adolescent, our society is enamored with the latest powerful technology, and perhaps somewhat contemptuous of our elders. But when we consider the whole of humanity, our culture is in its infancy, and needs to be more considerate and respectful of ancient knowledge. Many nurses today are making pilgrimages to other parts of the world, learning about healing modalities directly from the source.

Some are traveling to underdeveloped nations, bringing the best of our Western medicine and appropriate technology to share with those less fortunate. These nurses report that their hearts feel full, and they are grateful for the opportunity to expand their horizons as nurses. Once again, these vistas are open to us all.

As nurses, we can be more interesting by remembering that we are teachers, seekers of knowledge, and research. We must open our minds and stretch ourselves in all directions so as to broaden and solidify nursing's base and provide a more integrated framework for our services. Once we add this expanded concept to that of medicine, we are (together) providing more total care for our patients.

Not only are we providing better care for our patients when we expand our vision, but we are truly taking better care of ourselves. As nurses, we have often stuffed our feelings about the ways in which patients (and we) are treated. We have looked away or numbed ourselves in order to accommodate to the needs of the system.

Perhaps we have paid a steeper price than first imagined through our denial. Perhaps it is time for nurses to speak out courageously; to put the machines on the back shelf and use them only when necessary, and use them wisely. We must move forward in good conscience, with the knowledge that the welfare of consumers is our foremost responsibility.

A further thought to keep in mind: nurses can have miscar-

278

riages, doctors can have heart attacks . . . None of us is exempt from the frightening situations that plague the human population. We all need the peace of mind that comes from having spoken our truth and made a difference, and from protecting the rights of all people to receive safe, healing treatment.

A new era of health care is dawning. The time is now ripe for an expanded vision of the nurse: healer, health promoter, prevention specialist, health resource consultant, and wellness expert. Nurses involved in medicine's most technological advances can now add new tools to their repertoire to be even more effective. Nurses who wish to be back out in the community can begin to do so now. Nurse-run businesses are the wave of the future.

If the U.S. has consistently been willing to pay to educate more nurses during wartime, perhaps we can enlist government support to help us keep people well, and to stop the war against personal choice in health care. Many Americans suffer needlessly because they have no support system, no one to teach them about nutrition and hygiene, and no one to help them understand how they became sick, or addicted, in the first place. They need to learn how to handle these problems in the future.

A major increase in public health nursing could save millions of dollars in hospital fees. How tragic that we 'haven't had time' to provide some of the nurturing and education needed to decrease the overwhelming alienation responsible for so much of today's drug addiction and violence.

The Grandest Conspiracy

Nursing must now enlist the aid of consumers, politicians, allied health professionals, and technicians to rise and meet the crying need before us. We can join support with chiropractors, acupuncturists, nutritionalists, social workers, massage therapists, physical therapists, and those M.D.'s who are ready, so that we can all 'conspire' to bring more variety, choices, and nurturing back into health care.

A time of crisis is a perfect time for change. We must be creative in inspiring more nurses to enter the field, and more nurses to come back to the profession they left. When we inspire nursing to be a healthier place to work, many others will want to work alongside us.

We have thus far met the challenges of a demanding profession. Let us now turn on our creative and inspirational lights, shining over the entire medical system, washing away the impurities and illuminating that which is healthy.

Nursing is the unity of mind, body, and spirit on individual, family, and cultural levels. The vision for nursing's future is endless. You could be involved in environmental consultation, helping to monitor the resources carefully. You may, as Florence Nightingale did, become involved with the creation of health care facilities, from the ground up. Some of us will be out furthering the image of nursing in nursing schools, spreading new visions.

As we go about the joyful and endlessly creative task of revisioning nursing, we can adopt a humble spirit of gratitude. Now, finally, our time has come. Now we can easily perform our most exciting and heartfelt work. Renewed strength will arise from our minds and hearts, with compassion and healing as our shared goal.

Let us each inspire, conspire, and shine our lights into the world . . .

PART IV

A FUTURE VISION

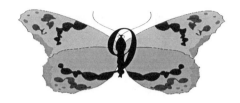

NURSING INSPIRES A HEALTH CARE REVOLUTION

A vision is a dream, a hope, a new way of seeing . . . Every nurse brings her own special vision to nursing. For some shared visions, see Visions of Nursing.[98] *Here, I share my vision. Soon, we will all be sharing our dreams together . . .*

It's a time to rejoice on planet Earth. Many diseases which once plagued and degraded human life have been eliminated. A great many hospitals have given way to healing centers all over the country. The remaining ones specialize in the treatment of the severely ill and trauma victims. Yet even within these existing hospitals and clinics, a healthy balance is maintained between technology and compassion, particularly in the Special Care Unit.

People from all walks of life have come to appreciate the importance of taking time to replenish the spirit - along with mind and body. Business professionals, parents, governmental leaders . . . all take regular time out here, anticipating their visits to this lovely environment much as people once embraced a long-awaited vacation.

The buildings are designed by the most humanistic architects available, with nursing's collaborative efforts. They are made of materials which resonate with the human energy field in the best possible way. The colors, aromas, sounds, and sights are likewise carefully chosen to induce deep relaxation.

Mr. Green is a business person, an average health care consumer. Years ago, he occasionally spent time in hospitals, receiving the highly technological treatments which were popular then. He was once operated on for a gall-bladder problem. Another time, he was hospitalized and monitored for cardiac arrhythmias. His daily life was moderately stressful, and he believed he was too busy to take time for himself.

Lately, thanks to the support and guidance of his nurse-advocate, he has become an avid recipient of the services offered in the Special Care Unit of his regular hospital. He can now make use of all the advances in cardiac medicine, while learning to care for himself simultaneously. If he did not have a medical condition, he would most likely partake of the retreat-type services offered in the new healing center nearby. For now, the Special Care Unit is the perfect solution.

This multi-disciplinary service, though once considered innovative, is now a standard practice in most hospitals. It is staffed by nurses who have been well-trained in the principles of health promotion. It is readily apparent that these nurses love their work, and seem to be energized by it. They obviously find it deeply satisfying to

286

teach people how to manage their health so as to stay out of the hospital more of the time. The nurses are private practitioners, hired as consultants to run the unit and oversee comprehensive care for each patient in a highly individualized manner.

Mr. Green checks in at the front desk. He is warmly received, as any traveler would be when he arrives exhausted at the front desk of a first class vacation resort. He is escorted, along with his personal belongings, to a peaceful room.

There he is cordially greeted by his caregiver, a nurse who will function as his personal health consultant. The room is comfortable in temperature, and he is oriented to his environment, then left alone to spend time in quiet reflection. Delicious, highly nourishing wholesome food, free of chemicals and preservatives, is available to him at all times. There is a range of services available, and he is invited to pick and choose among them, with the nurse's help. Together, they will devise a program consistent with his personal health goals, using in part the wealth of information available in books, audiotapes and video cassettes.

A team of licensed healers can be utilized as he desires. He can choose from physical therapy, acupuncture, massage and healing touch, music therapy, dance and movement therapy, guided imagery, psychotherapy, biofeedback, stretching and other forms of exercise. Were Mr. Green dying, he would have a specially-trained nurse available as his personal Life Transition Guide.

Many of these healing arts practitioners are also nurses who have broadened their concept of wellness through specializing in specific modalities. They often use hands-on approaches to stimulate the person's innate ability to heal himself. The air and water is pure and clean, and each person (client and staff alike) is made to feel

287

very special.

His visit is covered through his insurance and employee benefits. These corporations have come to understand that money is saved by investing in preventive care. They now appreciate the improvement in social problems that used to arise out of pervasive cultural dis-ease. In fact, there is general agreement now that people need high-quality health education from an early age to enhance their inner communications with themselves, and their external communications with others. The society now provides its citizens with health awareness education as one of the first things taught in school by nurse educators.

It is well-known that when a person has taken ample time inward and in health-promoting activities, that person is much more clear and effective in communications and work endeavors. There are health consultants, again often nurses, available to the person upon leaving a Special Care Unit. These nurse-guides assist in re-entry and also serve to promote health and well-being in the home and work environments.

These healers have become a vital link to their community, and to think some were once disgruntled nurses! Their dedicated commitment to the principles of health-maintenance made them instrumental in the formation of these new services. Thousands of 'lost' nurses (who had quit their profession during the 'handless/ heartless era') managed to create a place for themselves in the new health care system. Nursing, the key element of this humane new system, now commands great respect and appreciation, as well as financial remuneration. Their position is enviable, and is aspired to by a great many young people in their society. Those who practice outside the hospitals and healing centers likewise feel highly respected for their contributions.

The dream has come true. Many of the well-trained nurses who had abandoned their profession in disillusionment in the latter 20th-century have now come back in full force to play their crucial role in the newly-created model. Now, they can laugh about a time when it was unpopular to be a nurse.

There are also more who have seen these changes as an opportunity to joyfully honor their nurturing side as nurses. These men likewise provide gentle loving care to those who require a convalescence from the stresses of daily life. They are serving as role models for the man of the future, who is much more in touch with and accepting of his feminine side. They have discovered that they can be whole, healthy men, and need not abandon their masculinity to do loving work, nor ignore their feminine strength. Similarly, women understand that they don't have to try to be men to work with them. In fact, their feminine nature offers a pleasant balance, which is comfortably expressed in their lives and work. Now, without restraint, each is free to be the best person she or he can be.

It also became apparent that part of nursing's work was to be more politically assertive in decisions that affect our nation's health and well-being. Nursing's voice came through loud and clear, due to the conspiratorial efforts of a large number of nurses, supported by other practitioners and consumers. Another major change has occurred in the active guardianship of the planet's resources and ecology, inspired by conscientious and well-informed nursing leadership.

Now, nurses are on the vanguard of society, protecting the environment, and promoting conscious consumerism on many levels. We have acknowledged our true role as health educators, and serve on governmental committees in every part of the country and world. We made decisions not to allow reckless environmental accidents, or the inappropriate application of technology. We now serve as advisors on nuclear issues, recycling possibilities, and to industry regarding foods, medicinals, air and water quality, and health hazards.

Nursing has come a long way in a short time, having accepted the challenge of empowerment for ourselves, our clients, and our nation.

Yes, this is a high time in health care. Recovering our lost art was not accomplished overnight. It took the courage and dedication of many people, combining hearts, voices and skills, to effect a much-needed change. It was a movement started by nurses, and further strengthened by allied health professions. The consumers of health care were ripe and ready for empowerment. Doctors began to see the wisdom of supporting and respecting the other members of the health team, and it snowballed into a sweeping social movement which broke the old molds, allowing for upheaval. The Revolution in health care led to a strengthening of the fabric of society.

Many blessings came from that period of crisis and transition. It took thousands of nurses quitting, then patients and doctors likewise turning, disgusted, from an inhumane institutionalized system that served no one very well.

As they joined forces, each person was healed;

As they joined forces, each profession was healed;

As they joined forces, health care was transformed . . .

And each person had her own special role in . . .

The Nightingale Conspiracy.

EPILOGUE

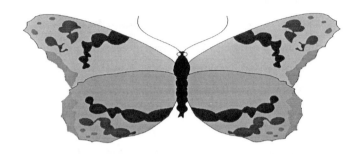

A New Era Dawns

We've all seen the modern medical symbol called a caduceus. It is a staff with two snakes intertwined. Back in the Days of Aesculapius, the symbol for the temples of healing was a staff with only one snake wrapped around it. People came to worship the god of good health, praying for forgiveness and relief.

In our country years ago, the U.S. Army Medical Corps decided to adopt this ancient symbol of healing, but some graphic artist made an error, and instead of having one snake around the staff, he drew two. This was not the symbol of Aesculapius, God of Healing. It was instead the symbol of Hermes, God of Commerce and Personal Gain!

Could this error explain some of the confusion in our present medical system? Perhaps so, for at an early stage in the development of our health care, we began to invoke the wrong deity. As a result, hospitals, administrators, drug companies, and doctors preside over

295

the booming business of commercial medicine. Is it not time for all of us to join forces and call strongly upon the more fundamental powers of Health and Healing - curing and caring?

A new era is dawning in medicine - *if, and only if,* we can each assume our most powerful position in the health care system. It is a time for more humane and compassionate health care. The nursing profession is preparing to assume a leadership role to usher in this exciting new age, and consumers need to be assertive to support these positive changes. Many have already begun the work.

This book is a 'call to arms' - for all caregivers - to promote more 'high touch' in our high-tech world, to *put more caring back into curing*, and to unite. Together, we will create a less costly, more healthy system - one that empowers us all.

REFERENCES/ENDNOTES

[1] Barbara Ehrenreich, and Diedre English, *Witches, Midwives & Nurses,* (New York: Feminist Press, 1973).

[2] Abraham Flexner, (Carnegie Foundation, 1910).

[3] Deepok Chopra, M.D., *Quantum Healing,* (New York: Bantam, 1989).

[4] Michael Brown, RN, *Nurses: The Human Touch*, New York: Ballantine, 1992).

[5] Ibid. pp. 286-288.

[6] Martha Rogers, Keynote Address: American Holistic Nurses Association National Conference (1992), Hot Springs, Arkansas.

[7] U.S. Government, Department of Health & Human Services, December 1988. Secretary's Commission on Nursing, Final Report, Volume I, Washington, D.C.

[8] Abraham Maslow, *Toward A Psychology of Being,* (New York: Van Nostrand Reinhold, 1969).

[9] M. Patricia Donahue, Ph.D., R.N., *Nursing: The Finest Art*, (St. Louis: C. V. Mosby Company, 1985).

[10] Florence Nightingale, "Cassandra", (England, 1852).

[11] Florence Nightingale, *Notes on Nursing: What It Is, and What It Is Not*, (London: Harrison & Sons, 1859).

[12] Ibid.

[13] Committee on the Grading of Nursing Schools, *Nursing, Patients, & Pocketbooks,* (1928).

[14] Isabel M. Stewart, letter to Lillian A. Hudson, c.1940-47 "Reminiscences of Isabel M. Stewart", (New York: Oral History Research Office, Columbia University, 1961).

[15] Donahue, Op. Cit., p. 445.

[16] John Bradshaw, *Bradshaw on the Family: A Revolutionary Way of Self-Discovery,* (Deerfield Beach, Florida: Health Communications, Inc., 1988).

[17] Anne Wilson Scaef, *When Society Becomes An Addict,* (New York: Harper & Row, 1987).

[18] Caryn Summers, R.N., *Caregiver, Caretaker: From Dysfunctional to Authentic Service in Nursing,* (Mt. Shasta: Commune-A-Key Publishing, 1992).

[19] Philip A. Kalisch, Ph.D. and Beatrice J., R.N., Ed.D., FAAN, *The Changing Image of the Nurse,* (Menlo Park, CA: Addison-Wesley Publishing Company, Health Science Division, 1992).

[20] Scott W. Shiffer, B.S.N., "Hollywood Nurses: A Muddled American Image", *California Nursing Review,* (Vol. 11, #3, May/June 1989).

[21] O. Carl Simonton, and J. Creighton, *Getting Well Again,* (Los Angeles: J.P. Tarcher, 1978).

[22] Joseph Campbell, *The Power of Myth,* (New York: Doubleday 1988).

[23] Geoffrey Cowley, *Newsweek,* (Oct. 19, 1992), p.74.

[24] Michio Mushi, *The Teachings of Michio Kushi,* (Boston: East West Foundation, 1972).

[25] Barbara M. Dossey, R.N., M.S. et al., *Holistic Nursing: A Handbook for Practice,* (Rockville, Md.: Aspen 1988).

[26] Lynn Keegan, R.N., Ph.D., "The History and Future of Healing" from *Holistic Nursing: A Handbook for Practice,* Dossey, et al., (Rockville, MD: Aspen Publications, 1988).

[27] Ibid. p.58

[28] Ibid. p.59

[29] Ibid. p.64

[30] Ibid.

[31] Ibid. p.65

[32] Ibid. p.64

[33] Ibid. p.65

[34] Flanders Dunbar, *Psychosomatic Diagnosis,* (New York: Paul B. Haeber, Inc., 1945).

[35] Hans Selye, *The Stress of Life,* (New York: McGraw-Hill, 1956).

[36] Thomas H. Holmes and Richard Rahe, "The Social Readjustment Rating Scale", *Journal of Psychosomatic Research* Vol. 11, (1967) pp. 213-218.

300

[37] Halbert L. Dunn, M.D., Ph.D., *High Level Wellness: A Collection of 29 Short Talks on Different Aspects of the Theme "High Level Wellness for Man & Society",* (Virginia: R.W. Beatty, Ltd., 1961).

[38] Mark LaLonde, *A New Perspective on the Health of Canadians,* (Ottawa: Government of Canada, 1974).

[39] U.S. Senate Select Committee on Nutrition and Human Needs, "Dietary Goals for the United States", (Washington, D.C.: U.S. Government Printing Office, 1977).

[40] Marilyn Ferguson, *The Aquarian Conspiracy,* (Los Angeles: J.P. Tarcher, Inc., 1980).

[41] Ibid., pp. 246-248.

[42] American Holistic Medical Association, 4101 Lake Boone Trail, Suite 201, Raleigh, North Carolina 27607.

[43] Nurse Healers Professional Associates, 175 Fifth Ave., #3399, New York, NY 10010.

[44] Ivan Illich, *Medical Nemesis: The Expropriation of Health,* (New York: Pantheon, 1976).

[45] Landrun B. Shettles, M.D., Ph.D. and David Rorvik, *How To Choose the Sex of Your Baby,* First Ed., (New York: Doubleday, 1984).

[46] Susan Faludi, *Backlash: The Undeclared War Against American Women,* (New York: Crown Publishers, 1991), p.430.

[47] Myra Stark, (author of Introduction to "Cassandra: Angry Outcry Against the Forced Idleness of Victorian Women, by F. Nightingale), (New York: Feminist Press, 1979), pp. 13-14.

[48] Keegan, Op. Cit. p. 65.

[49] Nightingale, Op. Cit. *Notes on Nursing,* pp. 2-4.

[50] Delores Krieger, Ph.D., *The Therapeutic Touch,* (Englewood Cliffs, NJ: Prentice-Hall, Inc., 1979).

[51] Marvin Belsky, M.D., *How To Choose and Use Your Doctor,* (New York: Arbor House, 1975).

[52] Ibid. p. 88.

[53] Ibid. pp. 102-103.

[54] Kahlil Gibran, *The Prophet,* (New York: Alfred A. Knopf, 1923), pp. 58-59.

[55] Robert S. DeRopp, *The Master Game,* (New York: Dell Publishing Co., 1968), p. 21.

[56] George Ohsawa, *Zen Macrobiotics,* (Boston: George Oshawa Foundation, 1965), p. 66.

[57] Moshe Feldenkrais, *Awareness Through Movement,* (New York: Harper & Row, 1972).

[58] Alexander Lowen, *The Betrayal of the Body,* (New York: Macmillan & Co., 1967).

[59] Daniela Gioseffi, *Earth Dancing: Mother Nature's Oldest Rite,* (Pacific Grove, CA: Artemis Imports Publishing, 1980).

[60] Erich Fromm, *The Art of Loving,* (New York: Bantam Books, 1963).

[61] Ibid., p. 50.

[62] Ashley Montague, *Touching,* (New York: Harper & Row, 1972).

[63] Sarah F. Hall, R.N., M.S.N. and Linda M. Wray, R.N., M.S.N., "Codependency: Nurses Who Give Too Much", *American Journal of Nursing,* Vol. 89, #11, pp. 1456-1460.

[64] Gladys Taylor McGarey, M.D., *Born To Live,* (Phoenix, Arizona: Gabriel Press, 1980).

[65] Margretta M. Styles, *On Nursing: Towards a New Endowment,* (St. Louis: C.V. Mosby Co., 1982), p. 8.

[66] David Willard, R.N., and Candace Snow, *I'm Dying To Take Care of You: Nurses & Codependence, Breaking the Cycles,* (Redmond, WA: Professional Counselor Books, 1989).

[67] Ibid., pp.3-4.

[68] Ibid.

[69] Summers, Op. Cit., p. 7.

[70] Ferguson. Op. Cit. p. 23.

[71] David Gershon, and Gail Straub, *Empowerment: The Art Of Creating Your Life As You Want It,* (New York: Dell Publishing Group, 1989), pp. 5-6.

[72] Albert Bandura, Ph.D., "Catecholamine Secretion as a Function of Perceived Coping Self-Efficacy, *Journal of Consulting and Clinical Psychology,* Vol. 53, #3, (1985), pp. 406-414.

[73] Victor Frankl, *Man's Search for Meaning,* (Boston: Beacon Press, 1959).

[74] Ibid., p.12.

[75] Bandura, Loc. Cit.

[76] Ibid., p. 407.

302

[77] Ibid.

[78] Albert Bandura, Ph.D. and Elizabeth Ozer, "Mechanisms Governing Empowerment Effects: A Self-Efficacy Analysis", *Journal of Personality & Social Psychology,* Vol. 58 (1990), p. 472.

[79] Ibid., pp. 472-486.

[80] Ibid., p. 486.

[81] Napoleon Hill, *Think and Grow Rich,* (New York: Ballantine Books, 1960).

[82] Ibid., p. 19.

[83] Ibid., p. 50.

[84] Ibid., pp. 75-76.

[85] Ibid., p. 100.

[86] Ibid., p. 103.

[87] Ibid., pp. 168-9.

[88] Ibid., p. 104.

[89] Ibid., p. 167.

[90] Ibid., pp. 105-6.

[91] Ibid., pp. 170-1.

[92] National Nurses in Business Association (NNBA), 1000 Burnett Ave., Suite 450, Concord, California, 94520, (510) 356-2642

[93] American Holistic Nurses Association (AHNA), 4101 Lake Boone Trail, Suite 201, Raleigh, North Carolina, 27607, (919) 787-5181

[94] Stephen R. Covey, *Principle-Centered Leadership,* (New York: Summit Books, 1990).

[95] Ibid. p. 17.

[96] Ibid. pp. 33-39.

[97] Laura Gasparis, R.N., M.A., CEN, CCRN and Joan Swirsky, R.N., M.S., CS, *Nurse Abuse: Impact and Resolution,* (New York: Power Publications, 1990).

[98] Charlotte McGuire, R.N., M.A., *Vision of Nursing,* (Raleigh, NC: American Holistic Nurses Association/Light Technology Publishing, 1989).

RECOMMENDED READING

I personally have found the following books to be of great value in relation to the topics of empowerment, women's issues, holistic health, and nursing.

Acterberg, Jeanne. *Woman As Healer.* Boston: Shambhala, 1990.

Anderson, Sherry Ruth and Patricia Hopkins. *The Feminine Face of God.* New York: Bantam, 1991.

Ashley, Jo Ann. *Hospitals, Paternalism, and the Role of the Nurse.* Teachers College, Columbia University, 1976.

Beattie, Melody. *Codependent No More.* New York: Harper & Row, 1987.

Carson, Verna Benner, R.N., M.S. *Spiritual Dimensions of Nursing Practice.* Philadelphia: W. B. Saunders Company, 1989.

Castine, Jacqueline. *Recovery from Rescuing.* Deerfield Beach, Florida: Health Communications, Inc., 1989.

Chenevert, Melodie, R.N., B.A., M.S. *STAT: Special Techniques in Assertiveness Training.* St. Louis: C.V. Mosby, 1989.

Clements, Imelda and E. Jane Martin. *Nursing and Holistic Wellness.* Dubuque, Iowa: Kendall/Hunt Publishing Co., 1990.

Donahue, M. Patricia, Ph.D., R.N. *Nursing: The Finest Art.* St. Louis, MO: C.V. Mosby, Inc., 1985.

Dossey, Barbara M., R.N., M.S., et al. *Holistic Nursing.* Rockville, Maryland: Aspen, 1988.

Dossey, Larry M.D. *Beyond Illness*. Boston: Shambhala, 1984.

Duerk, Judith. *Circle of Stones*. San Diego, CA: LuraMedia, 1989.

Eichenbaum, Luise and Susie Orbach. *Between Women*. New York: Penguin Books, 1987.

Ehrenreich, Barbara and Deirdre English. *Witches, Midwives and Nurses*. New York: Feminist Press, 1973.

Faludi, Susan. *Backlash*. New York: Crown Publishers, 1991.

Ferguson, Marilyn. *The Aquarian Conspiracy*. Los Angeles, CA: J.P. Tarcher, Inc., 1980.

Gasparis, Laura R.N., M.A., CEN, CCRN and Joan Swirsky R.N., M.S., CS(ed.). *Nurse Abuse*. New York: Power Publications, 1990.

Gershon, David & Gail Straub. *Empowerment*. NewYork: Dell, 1989.

Gioseffi, Daniela. *Earth Dancing*. Pacific Grove, CA: Artemis Imports, 1980/1991.

Jacobson, Sharol F. R.N., Ph.D. and H. Marie McGrath R.N., Ph.D., (ed.). *Nurses Under Stress*. New York: John Wiley & Sons, 1983.

Kramer, Marlene R.N., Ph.D. *Reality Shock: Why Nurses Leave Nursing*. St. Louis, MO: C.V. Mosby Co., 1974.

Kraegel, Janet R.N. and Mary Kachoyeanos, R.N. *"Just A Nurse"*. New York: E.P. Dutton/Penguin, 1989.

Leonard, Linda. *The Wounded Woman*. Boulder: Shambala, 1983.

Lerner, Harriet Goldhor Ph.D. *The Dance of Anger*. New York: Harper & Row, 1985.

McGarey, Gladys T. *Born To Live*. Phoenix: Gabriel Press,

306

1980.

Murdock, Maureen. *The Heroine's Journey*. Boston: Shambhala, 1990.

McGuire, Charlotte R.N., M.A.,(ed.). *Visions of Nursing*. Sedona, AZ: Light Technology Publishing, 1989.

National Nurses in Business Association. *How I Became A Nurse Entrepeneur*. Petaluma, CA: NNBA, 1991.

Phelps, Stanlee M.S.W. & Nancy Austin, M.B.A. *The Assertive Woman*. San Luis Obispo, CA: Impact Publishers, 1975/1987.

Rossman, Martin M.D. *Healing Yourself*. New York: Walker & Co., 1987.

Smythe, Emily E.M.. *Surviving Nursing*. Menlo Park, CA: Addison-Wesley Publishing Co., Nursing Division, 1984.

Schaef, Anne Wilson. *Women's Reality*. New York: Harper & Row, 1981/1985.

Summers, Caryn R.N. *Caregiver, Caretaker*. Mt. Shasta, CA: Commune-A-Key Publishing, 1992.

Snow, Candace and David Willard R.N. *I'm Dying to Take Care of You*. Redmond, WA: Professional Counselor Books, 1989.

Steinem, Gloria. *Revolution from Within*. Boston: Little, Brown, and Company, 1992.

Shames, Richard M.D. and Chuck Sterin, M.S., Ph.D. *Healing with Mind Power*. Emmaus, PA: Rodale Press, 1978.

Wegscheider-Cruse, Sharon. *The Miracle of Recovery*. Deerfield Beach, FL.: Health Communications, Inc., 1989.

The author welcomes any feedback or responses to *The Nightingale Conspiracy,* but regrets that she may not be able to respond to every contact.

Karilee Halo Shames, R.N., Ph.D.
c/o Nurse Empowerment Workshops
PO Box 2398
Mill Valley, CA. 94942

INDEX

M

Maslow   24, 222
medicine man   96, 97, 100, 113
meditation   81, 86, 162, 164, 167, 178, 179, 180, 184, 205, 206, 214,
          218, 222, 225
mentor   229, 252
midwifery 13, 68, 69, 70, 87, 161, 165, 166, 167, 170, 171, 174,
          175, 240
mindpower   15, 277
movement 13, 19, 37, 49, 76, 151, 209, 210- 212, 214, 236, 256,
          287, 290
mythology   49, 62, 63, 143

N

nacebo effect   16
Nightingale   19, 24, 31, 33, 39, 45, 51, 119, 127, 183, 185, 228,
          232, 235, 240, 271, 275, 280, 291
Nurses in Transition   17, 63, 256
nutrition 19, 58, 79, 86, 151, 209, 228, 231, 279, 280

P

paradigm   150, 151, 152, 154, 191, 236, 244
paradigm shift   19, 189
prevention   10, 153, 157
preventive   61, 113, 247, 272, 276, 279, 288

R

recovery 16, 40, 48, 59, 60, 61, 67, 68, 217, 218, 236, 243
revolution   39, 150, 275, 285, 290
rituals 74, 95, 96, 97, 212

.... **THE NIGHTINGALE CONSPIRACY**
IS GROWING.

IF YOU ARE INSPIRED
TO CONSPIRE MORE:

N.E.W.S.
P.O. BOX 2398
Mill Valley, CA 94942
415-388-NEWS
800-366-NEWS

Please stay in touch. Fill out the information below, and you will be put on the mailing list for all upcoming Nightingale Conspiracy events and publications.

Name_____

Address_____

City, State, Zip_____

Phone(s): Day (____)_____ Eve (____)_____

Places of Work_____
(Could they benefit from a Nurse Empowerment Workshop? If so, please fill out)

Inservice Director_____

Facility Name_____

Complete Address_____

City, State, Zip_____

Phone (   ) _____

Also - Are you interested in:

Contributing your story for a book? _____

Sponsoring a Healing Movement Workshop? _____

Attending Mother/Daughter Healing retreat? _____

Subscribing to Nightingale Networking Newsletter? _____

Promoting the sales of this book? _____

Attending Nightingale Conspiracy Retreat? _____

Mail to: NEWS, P.O. Box 2398, Mill Valley, CA 94942
Phone: (415) 388-NEWS or (800) 366-NEWS
(PLEASE USE OTHER SIDE OF PAGE FOR COMMENTS)

A Note from the Publisher

We hope you have enjoyed *The Nightingale Conspiracy.* We are extremely pleased to have published it, and to play a part in the 'Conspiracy'. It has truly been an inspired journey. If you wish additional copies of *The Nightingale Conspiracy,* please send your check in the amount of $19.95 for each copy ordered plus $3.00 shipping per total order to:

Healthcare Management Innovations
484 Bloomfield Avenue
Montclair, New Jersey 07042

Healthcare Management Innovations, under its imprints **Enlightenment Press** and **HMI Press**, publishes books of interest and importance to the nursing community and the general public. We welcome queries and manuscripts in the areas of Healthcare, Holistic and General Nursing Issues, Spirituality, NDE's and other closely related topics. Please send with SASE to the above address.

If you would like to receive a copy of our catalog, *Nursing Evolution,* which features books and tapes in the above areas, please call (201) 746-0977.

ß